RAQUEL
WINNER OF THE FIRST AMERICAN HEALTH BOOK AWARDS

"Are you in great shape and want to stay that way, but you're looking for a method to maintain your high standards? Then I wrote this book for you.

"Are you almost in great shape, but not quite, and looking for that extra something that allows you to make the grade? Then I wrote this book for you, too.

"Or have you gotten to the point where you're just fed up—you've never been in great shape—and you wish this whole fitness craze would dry up and blow away? Then I wrote this book especially for you."

RAQUEL

"To preserve her famous curves, Welch has tried jogging, aerobics, and weight lifting. Then she discovered Hatha Yoga, an experience she describes as 'when East meets Welch.'"

People

"MORE THAN JUST ANOTHER CELEBRITY HOW-TO. IT HAS CHARM AND HUMOR."

Ladies Home Journal

"RAQUEL gives readers a very intimate look at the lady herself...because she talks in simple language about simple problems and situations that affect lots of women."

Fit Magazine

"THE APPROACH IS NO NONSENSE AND RAQUEL ENCOURAGES THE READER WITH STORIES OF HER OWN STRUGGLES."

USA Today

"FABULOUS ADVICE! Follow Raquel's unbeatable exercise regimen, and glean invaluable tips on nutrition, style, clothes, makeup, hair!"

Cosmopolitan

To André, my husband, my lover, my friend.

A Fawcett Columbine Book

Published by Ballantine Books

Copyright © 1984 by Raquel Welch

Grateful acknowledgment is made for permission to reprint the following:
Spinal Chart by permission of Sinel Publishing Inc.
Food Combining chart by Dr. James D'Adamo, Toronto.
Wonder Soup recipe from *Natural Way to Sexual Health* by Henry G. Bieler. Copyright © 1972, by permission of Charles Publishing Company.
The slogan "Food Is Your Best Medicine" from *Food Is Your Best Medicine* by Henry G. Bieler. Copyright © 1982 by Ballantine Books, a division of Random House, Inc.
Excerpt from *Doing It with Style* by Quentin Crisp and Donald Carroll. Copyright © 1981 by Carroll Regnier Assoc., Inc. Used by permission of Franklin Watts Inc.
The following are claimed trademarks and service marks of RWP, Inc.:
Total Beauty, Active Relaxation, and Organic Feedback.
A list of photo credits can be found on page 264.

Library of Congress Catalog Card Number: 85-47665

ISBN: 0-449-90169-6

Manufactured in the United States of America

First Ballantine Books Trade Edition: February 1986

10 9 8 7 6 5 4 3 2 1

RAQUEL

THE RAQUEL WELCH
TOTAL BEAUTY AND FITNESS
PROGRAM

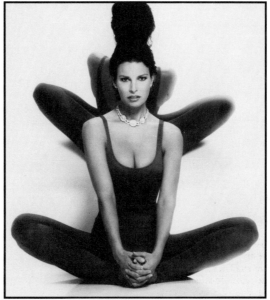

PHOTOGRAPHS
BY ANDRE WEINFELD

Fawcett Columbine
New York

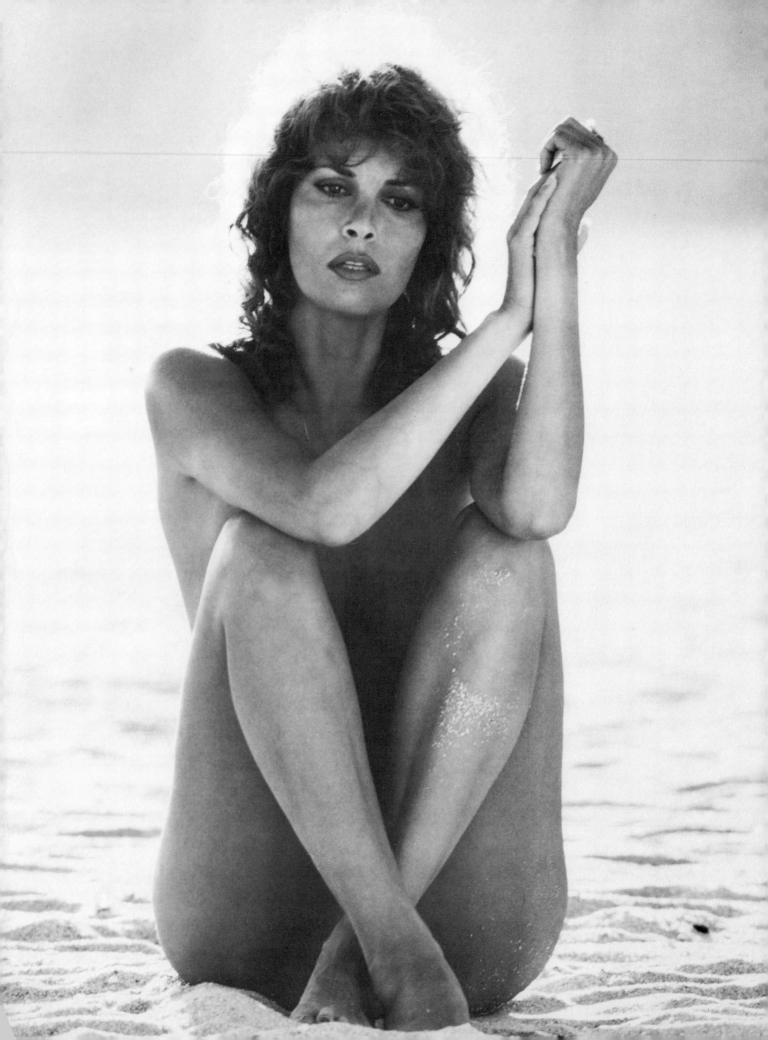

My body is the shape I live in,
and it shapes the way I live.

R.W.

CONTENTS

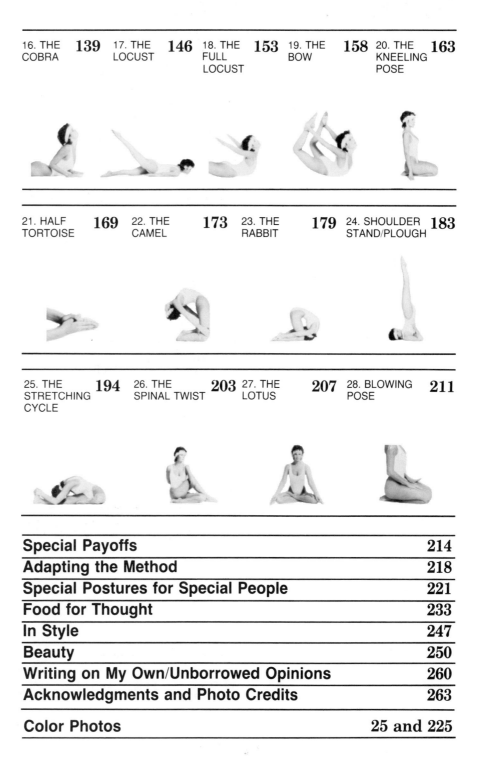

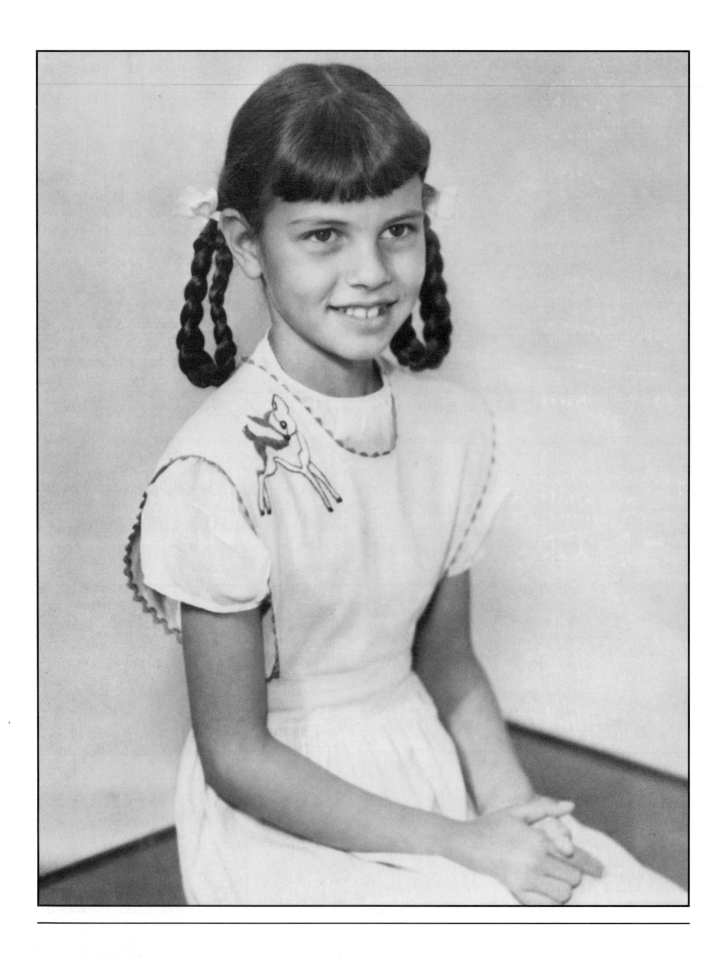

Introduction

The inspiration for this book goes back seven years, when I discovered a method of physical fitness called Hatha Yoga, a method that not only satisfied my need to stay in shape, but also created new untapped resources of energy and creativity in me that until then I didn't even know existed.

The Source

Hatha Yoga, practiced in India for centuries, is to physical activities what Latin is to many languages. As you read through these pages, therefore, you'll be able to recognize the origins of the push-up, of modern-dance stretches, acrobatics, gymnastics, and ballet positions, among others. So if your goal is *total* beauty and fitness, why not go straight to the source?

The Best of Both Worlds

Let me make it clear, however, that this method is not your average, run-of-the-mill Hatha Yoga routine. It's quite different from the yoga offered in most classes that teach the subject. For one thing, it's quite strenuous and therefore it stimulates swift and remarkable physical results. Although engineered to suit the

Opposite: *At seven years old, total beauty meant only one thing to me—that the braided loops would have to go!*

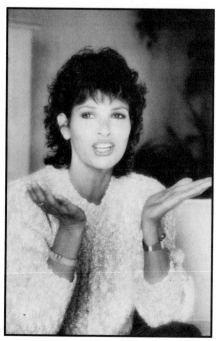

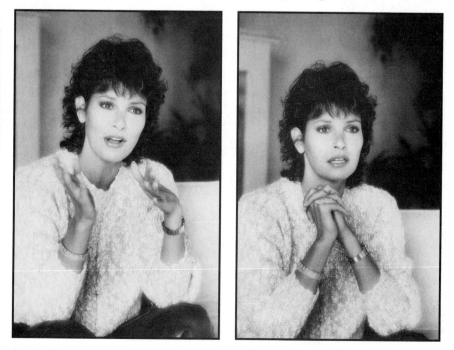

Western mentality, it does not violate the principles of yoga. It's both nonviolent and physically aggressive, so it combines the best of both worlds.

Mind and Body

The program illustrated in these pages should not be confused with what I call the "fitness fallout." It's not beauty "tips" and "hints," it is a bona fide, complete fitness program consisting of twenty-eight separate postures scientifically designed to work 100 percent of your mind and body.

The fact is that the mind and body are interrelated—they never stop interacting. Everything we think and feel is related to our physical form and the shape that form is in. Since the physical and mental aspects of each of us are inseparable, why embark on a program that concerns itself only with outward appearances?

The Shape We Live In . . .

Nevertheless, as we all know, externals *do* govern our lives—for better or for worse. There are times when we all feel trapped by our physical forms, convinced we've inherited shapes that perform poorly to our will and don't express our true nature. We're stuck inside our bodies every day, trying to make the best of the situation. Some of us even try to forget we have a body at all; but if we don't take care of it, it will start acting up on us like a neglected child. That's why I find the only time I can "forget" mine is *after* I've taken care of it. Then and only then am I free to escape

The fact is that the mind and body are interrelated—they never stop interacting.

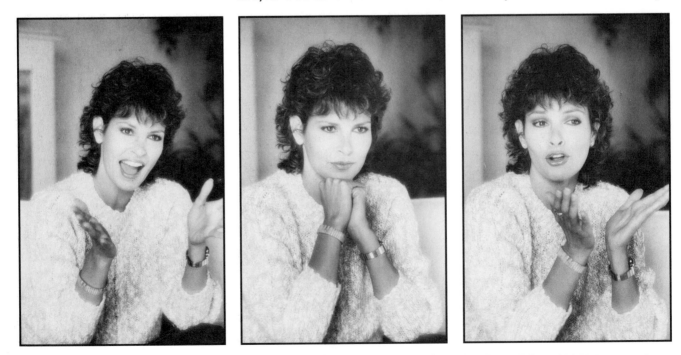

the physical, and let my mind settle on other, more engaging things. That's why the system we use as a springboard for this freedom is so important . . . and why I've chosen this method of Hatha Yoga.

. . . Shapes the Way We Live

Through the practice of this daily routine, I've come to realize that not only is my body the shape I live in, but it also shapes the *way* I live. I find it ironic that even though I live inside my body—through my body, with it, and because of it—it took this age-old method to make me aware of something so self-evident. Yet it's something we all tend to forget. This system acts as a constant reminder of that fact. It *insures* that we stay in sync—and makes us better able to absorb the punches that life throws our way.

The Best You've Ever Felt

The method I've presented in this book is for all ages and sexes, but especially for those thousands of women who, over the years, all around the world, have stopped me on a street corner or written letters asking, "What do you do to look the way you do?"

Now, of course, I'm not promising that if you follow this method you'll end up looking like me (wouldn't that be boring?), but I can guarantee that you'll look the best you've ever looked—and, more important, *be* at your best both mentally and physically. You'll start to feel so good in your own skin that you won't want to change places with anyone else.

We all feel trapped by our physical forms, convinced we've inherited shapes that perform poorly to our will and don't express our true nature.

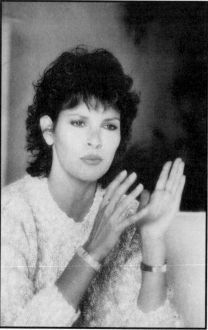
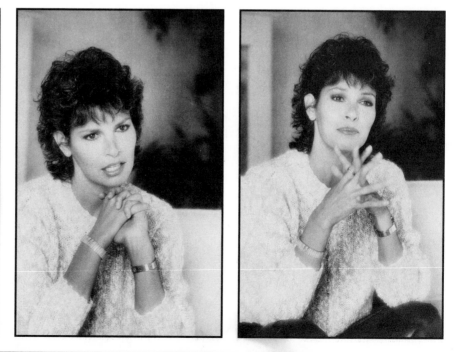

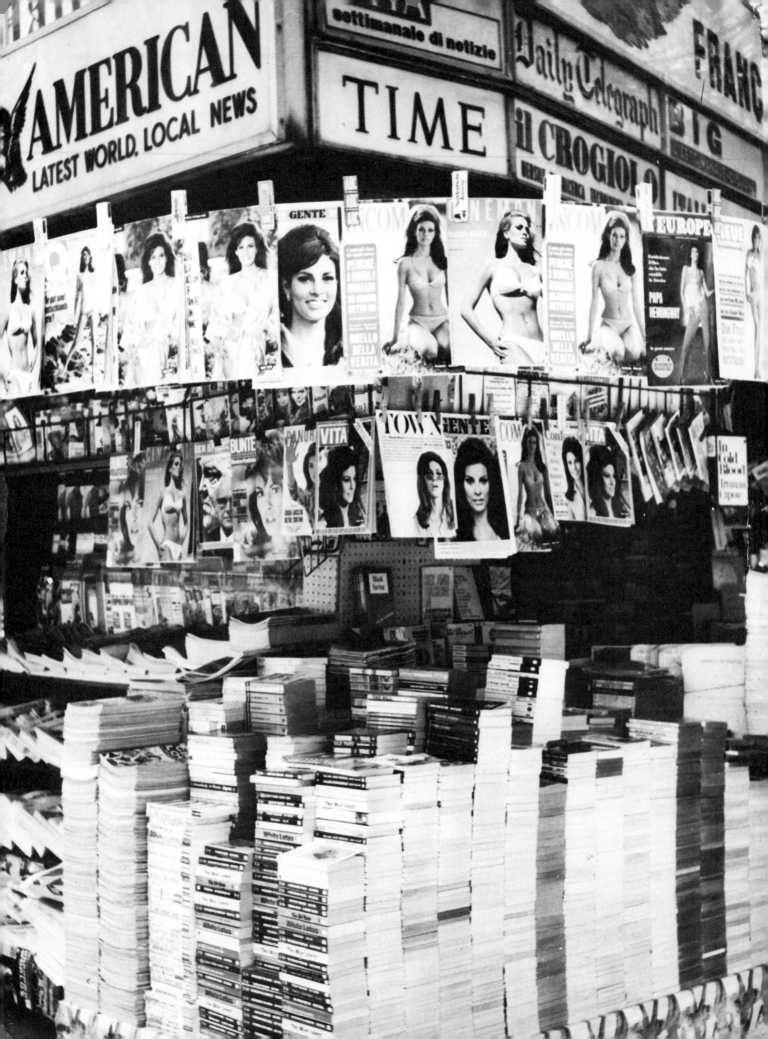

Search for the Answers

As an actress, I've struggled all my life to find that point of equilibrium in which, as an American girl, I could find happiness in the precarious balance between "making it" in the system (read: "Success" with a capital S) and making it with myself (read: happiness and peace of mind).

Before I started to practice this method, I often found myself frazzled from the demands of my work schedule, from the pressures of being in the public eye, and generally from living in a fishbowl where my every word and gesture were repeated. How to get off the roller coaster . . . how to perform for the public and yet take control of my own destiny, how not to panic? These were the questions I asked myself a hundred times over. It was, to say the least, debilitating.

Nirvana Anna

It was in pursuit of this golden land of "no panic"—when all around me were the echoes of flattery and insult, encouragement and disaster—that I began to think of myself as "Nirvana Anna"— the girl whose quest for peace of mind and harmony in the land of hype would know no bounds.

Because to catch the gold ring . . . to find the pot of riches at the end of the American rainbow, turns out to be a booby prize (no pun intended) without it. Ah, but where there's a will, there's a way. No jumping off buildings, no overdoses, and no hollow-eyed stares from drugs. I had two children at an early age and I felt I owed them, if nothing else, an example of *how not to trash yourself* when the going gets rough.

So here's Ms. Nirvana Anna trotting through the woods of trends, surrounded by the signposts of est, primal scream therapy, coffins full of water, the fruit-and-nuts group, the pseudo-intellectuals, the political activists, the cokeheads, the WASPs and aristocrats, the existentialists and the physical culturists, the macho men and the facho chicks, the squeaky cleans and the Europeans, the dingbats young and old, and, of course, since I'm an actress, "Hollywood"! Oh, the spirit is strong, but the flesh grows weak!

I had two children at an early age and I felt I owed them, if nothing else, an example of *how not to trash yourself* when the going gets rough.

Opposite: *"Making it": A fishbowl where my every word and gesture were repeated (Rome, 1968).*

Is it any wonder that in such an atomosphere I became somewhat discouraged, confused, and downright fed up? "Stop," I wanted to cry. "Shut up, will you, with your never-ending rap, on everything from macrobiotic diets to transcendental meditation, and your incessant dialogue on fitness and body building. . . . Just shut up!"

There's a point in the center of a hurricane where all is calm—an empty place at the vortex of all activity where nothing interferes. That's the place Nirvana Anna was looking for—that I was looking for—and I found it.

East Meets Welch

When my friend B.J. first mentioned yoga, it went in one ear and out the other. I had a built-in resistance to it. First, I didn't associate it in my mind with physical fitness—too passive was my hunch—and I had no intention of wandering around the hills of Hollywood in saffron robes. That was the image I had of yoga. Like most people, I had it lumped together in my mind with all things I considered mysteriously Eastern. Was it a sect? Was it a swami? Was it superweird?

After scanning the pages of the "Pretzel Books," I had been over- or *under*-whelmed by the assortment of every conceivable contortion in yogic history laid end to end before my very eyes. If it didn't bring to mind the prospect of wading barefoot through a sea of rubber bands, it would certainly scare anyone half to death!

Since then I've come to understand that what my friend was suggesting was a different kind of *Hatha Yoga*, a purely physical practice that is not at all passive, meditative, or mystical in nature.

3,000 Years B.C.

Developed some five thousand years ago in India, Hatha Yoga is the oldest existing physical-culture system in the world. In Sanskrit, *ha* means "sun," *tha* means "moon," and *yoga* means "to join together," in perfect harmony.

It was discovered that the body (the sun) and mind (the moon) could interact more freely if people weren't distracted by aches, pains, and stiffness. Nope, nothing superweird here. . . .

Nothing to Lose

But, thank God, B.J. didn't insist or try to convince me. I guess, deep down, I was afraid that yoga was some kind of cult;

I had no intention of wandering around the hills of Hollywood in saffron robes.

Below: *Back in One Million Years* B.C., *yoga hadn't been invented yet. But in this 1967 poster the natives seemed to be in pretty good shape.*

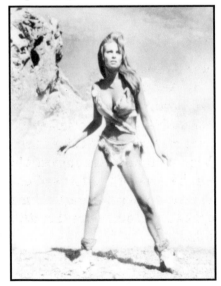

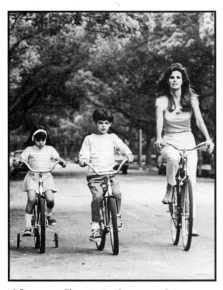

Above: *I've tried everything to stay in shape. Bicycling with my daughter, Tahnee, and my son, Damon, in 1969. Today, we all practice yoga.*

I don't want to Om-m-m out! . . . I'm a practical American girl; transcendental meditation makes me hostile!

and I didn't want to be converted. Since I'm a liberal and, more importantly, an individual, I've always loathed anything that has you pledging allegiance, taking an oath, or marching in step, so I was poised waiting for my friend to be more dogmatic. But she wasn't. Secretly, I was impressed.

My concerns, mind you, were not all so esoteric—I was interested in keeping my "well-publicized" body in shape. I'd been through every fitness trend from jogging to aerobics, from weight-lifting machines to home instructors and make-it-up-as-you-go routines, all to no avail. Rock music for exercise always jolted me too violently from a dead start into rhythms not of my own making. I tried to work up enthusiasm for facing a room filled with an army of chrome-plated machines, but it didn't take; it left me cold. I know some people like it, but—bottom line—it was not for me.

By this time I was ready—more than ready—for my friend's suggestion! I felt I'd seen it all, so what did I have to lose?

The First Time

The first time I walked into a yoga class, seven years ago, I thought, What am I doing here? I don't want to Om-m-m out! . . . I'm a practical American girl; transcendental meditation makes me hostile! That's exactly how I felt, as faces turned to look at me, check me out, size me up, and worst of all, recognize me.

I said to myself, Okay, I'm here: I may as well see it through. But my critical Virgo nature wasn't convinced. I was extremely skeptical of this whole "mysto," slightly esoteric, Eastern approach that was vaguely reminiscent of the Sixties, the Beatles, and the Maharishi. . . . Maybe I shouldn't stay after all, I hate incense—it makes me sneeze. But I did.

Three Feet off the Ground

Actually, there was no incense and no hocus-pocus either. The teacher, Bikram Choudhury, began the class with a series of strenuous standing poses, followed by floor postures to strengthen the spine and work the back of the torso. Although I experienced no pain, I was breathing hard and at times my muscles trembled with the effort. It wasn't easy, but even the poses that looked impossible also seemed attainable with practice, because of the focus of energy in the routine. The beauty and grace of the poses inspired me to try harder, and every time I thought I'd run out of gas (breath), the sequence would change to revitalize me.

By the end of my first class, I was walking three feet off the ground. I felt buoyant and in a wildly expansive mood. I flew home,

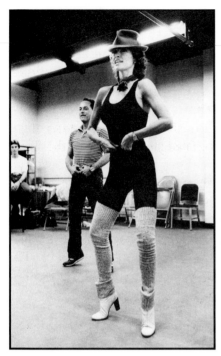

Above: *In rehearsal for* Woman of the Year, *with choreographer Tony Charmoli.*

where I tried to put a cap on my good spirits. Since I'd left that morning in a blue funk, I didn't want to alarm the natives; sometimes the laid-back level of activity in So. Cal. is not ready for such a spontaneous burst of high energy.

The Taj Mahal

I was having some difficulty containing myself because, as so often happens when you come upon some unexpected piece of good news, I was dying to share it with everyone in sight. You have to understand that for someone with a chronic case of low blood pressure and a tendency toward "Mediterranean anemia" (that's what they call it!), this newly found source of energy was a major triumph. It felt something like being presented with the key to the Taj Mahal.

RW's RPMs

I don't want to destroy your illusions about me, but for the most part I see myself as a well-proportioned wimp. Not only do I need help opening jam and pickle jars, but revolving doors do not respond to my push. Most of the rigors of early-morning rising for films, the horseback riding for Westerns, the roller-skating stunts, and the dance rehearsals on Broadway or for my nightclub shows, have been acts of will for me, rather than a smooth-going, well-oiled routine. It has always taken me a long time to get my RPMs revved up. Once they're running I'm alright, but what a ruthless struggle it used to be just to get my engines going.

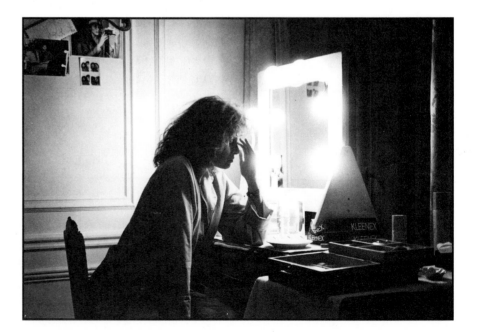

Right: *Any illusions of glamour in the movies are shattered by those 5:00* A.M. *makeup calls (Paris, 1976).*

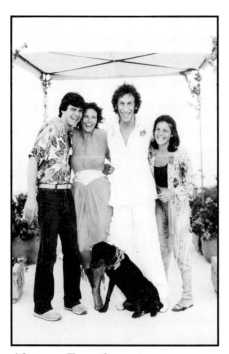

Above: *Together at my wedding, Baja, Mexico, 1980: Damon, me, André, Tahnee, and our dog, Chat.*

The Real Thing

Now, out of the blue, after so much resistance on my part, I'd stumbled on something called Hatha Yoga that woke me up physically and mentally and put me on track. I hoped it wasn't beginner's luck, because nothing other than a stiff cup of European-blend coffee had ever given me such a lift before. I decided not to shout the news. . . . I'd wait and see. Was this a flash in the pan, or was it the real thing?

Seven years later, I'm happy to report that it was the real thing. In other words, after a long search, I had finally and gratefully come to my journey's end. No more visions of overweight and poorly motivated health buffs chewing gum and reading paperback novels atop their exercycles. That was behind me now. I'd found the answer, the all-in-one approach that I'd adopt as my method.

Making It with Myself

Now I feel more centered. Various assaults on my nervous system seem to roll off my back and into perspective. I'm really no different from you—I have day-to-day problems, and all is not smooth as silk. But I am much better equipped, since doing yoga, to perform as an actress, have a loving and exciting marriage, deal with my children, make public appearances, see my friends, run my production company, and . . . write a book!

Sometimes I feel I could buckle under the weight of the pressure, but I've been able to rise to the challenge on most occasions without cracking. I've found reserves of energy and insight that I didn't know existed, but I've also learned when to stop. Sometimes the old siren call of "Everybody's doin' it" is pretty persuasive, but the fear of missing out on something doesn't seduce me into competing with anyone other than myself.

A New Approach

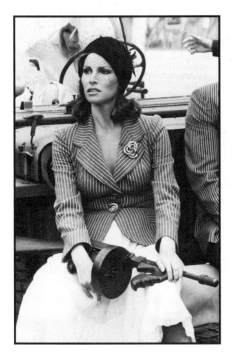

Above: *I didn't always use a cannon to kill a flea. Here, in the French film* L'Animal, *I only used a machine gun.*

Yoga represented a new approach for me. The first thing that attracted me to it was the virtual absence of pain.

No Pain

I've never been a stranger to pain—or afraid of it. I have suffered innumerable injuries on both stage and screen. In *Woman of the Year,* on Broadway, I dislocated my back, pulled my hamstring, and chipped a bone. The film *Kansas City Bomber,* for which I had to learn professional roller-skating in three weeks, left me with a broken wrist, a split lip, and a wrecked trapezius. And during the shooting of *The Legend of Walks Far Woman* for NBC Television, I pulled my Achilles tendon. The list goes on. . . .

Sometimes my enthusiasm for perfection caused me to suffer various physical and emotional discomforts unnecessarily. I could—and perhaps should—have used a stunt-double more often in my movies, but something usually impelled me to do it myself. Well, generosity of spirit is a good quality, but I got carried away with it. I always used a cannon to kill a flea. It's a quality in my nature, very useful in comedy acting, but in practical matters, it left me dissatisfied, because the rewards were almost never worth the monumental effort. So I don't pay homage to blind effort anymore. It's a no-win situation. Enough is enough and it always will be.

The Dynamic Duo

But, you may ask, how can I accomplish anything without pain and strain? This "dynamic duo" has become so familiar to us that the thought of giving them up is tantamount to sacrilege—to say nothing of the Guilt.

What about those Puritan voices inside shouting, "Pain is good for you. . . . If it doesn't hurt, it's not working. . . ." Well, I'm here to tell you they're wrong. Effort and pain are not the same thing. Pain, in fact, is energy spent in the wrong way, and there's enough of it in the world without the self-inflicted variety.

This method doesn't ask that you become a masochist. It just asks for your honest effort. Go as far as you can on any given day—*right up to the threshold of discomfort*—and hold the positions there. Each *consecutive* day, the threshold will be higher. Consistency is your friend when it comes to discomfort; every practice session literally chases the pain away.

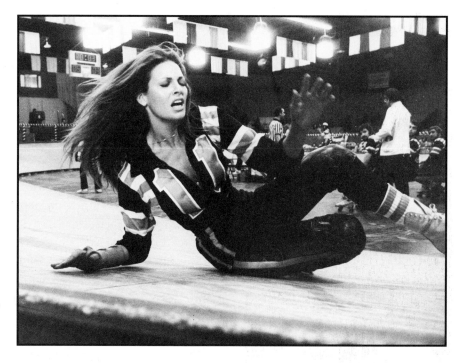

Right: *I've never been a stranger to pain or afraid of it. In* Kansas City Bomber *(1972), I performed many of my own stunts. Ouch!*

Below: *The trigger-happy syndrome—in* Hannie Caulder *(1972), I played a female gunslinger in search of her blue jeans.*

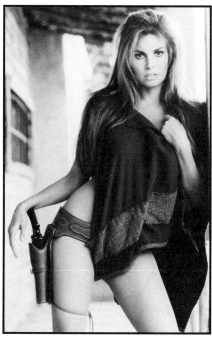

No Strain

You don't need to strain or force your body in this method. The goal implicit in each posture is enough for the moment. Outside elements may "force you to force" yourself in daily life. But you're released from that obligation here. The best thing is that this routine provides enough results to keep your effort at exactly the right level needed—no more, no less.

To strain is to push something past its limits. It can be described as a product of impatience. We force ourselves because we're not willing to wait, thereby causing unnecessary pain and injury. It's odd that when things develop naturally of their own accord one would seek to force the situation. Often, too, the misuse of force comes just when the goal is in sight—the old trigger-happy syndrome.

Meanwhile, who needs a wrenched back, a pulled tendon, and a limp? Physical fitness is supposed to improve your condition, not add insult to misery.

In any physical activity—even walking or riding a bicycle—there is some chance of injury. However, if you follow the instructions in this program carefully, the risk is slight. Nonetheless, check first with your physician if you have special health problems (such as a heart condition or extreme overweight); or in the case of a bad back, get the advice of your chiropractor.

Exercise is generally beneficial—and preferable to sedentary habits—especially under the supervision of a qualified instructor.

Haste Makes Waste

Yoga is the perfect example of that old Latin motto *festina lente,* or "make haste slowly." It makes the point that time well spent is worth a hundred times over what can be achieved in haste.

I like to say that fast bodies are like fast food: you don't have to wait, but you sacrifice quality and suffer afterward from a case of indigestion.

Nonetheless, most of us still rush around in ever-increasing circles as though speed were of the essence. Which leads me to suspect that, if one had to choose between doing things the "fast way" *with* pain, or doing things more slowly *without* pain, by and large we'd choose the former.

But easy come, easy go. If you throw yourself into any activity carelessly, the benefits are short-lived, and, also, you run the risk of injury. Why? Because when your body moves too swiftly, the momentum often carries it over the threshold of pain and results in a strained muscle. Then you lose valuable time . . . which was the whole reason for doing things fast in the first place. Haste makes waste—trite but true.

This routine encourages people to set their own pace and to avoid comparing themselves with others.

This routine encourages people to set their own pace and to avoid comparing themselves with others. It isn't a contest, after all. It's not *how many* you can do, but how many you can do *properly.* Why not work within your own limits, instead of somebody else's, and still achieve remarkable results? Improvement will be swift and the rewards almost immediate—they pile up faster than pennies in a jar—only the approach is gradual and meticulous.

Listen to your body rhythms, be a spectator to your own progress—and watch what happens!

Inner Dialogue

Below: *Inner dialogue: taking a look at yourself, eye to eye— getting to know yourself and what makes you tick.*

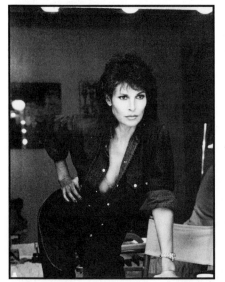

Every day we bypass—or simply don't recognize—messages sent by the body which try to signal us that our needs are not being met, or that we are overindulging. Hatha Yoga is the perfect tool to help you identify these signals. It will remove you from outside interference and provide you with an oasis where you can hear yourself think and feel. This is what "inner dialogue" is all about. Your ability to listen and interpret that dialogue is indispensable. It's the key to your health.

In practice, it will be impossible to bypass these signals and still do the postures correctly, thereby *insuring* that those *body signals* get through.

For example, as you go along, you will come to recognize points of tension and stiffness in your body as more than just telltale signs of physical inflexibility. These tension points are also indications of *mental or emotional stiffness*—including the rigidity of a closed mind!

Overflexibility, on the other hand, signals something quite different. It indicates a *need* for building strength—both physically *and* mentally. Your flexibility may allow you to perform the postures beautifully, to the envy of others; but the difficulty arises when it comes to *holding* the position for the full count. *Holding and staying is how you build strength* in Hatha Yoga. So if you have difficulty here, perhaps it means that you need a firm resolve in your daily life and are therefore too accommodating and easily taken advantage of.

The strength you build through this method correlates *directly* with your ability to assert yourself with confidence in your daily life.

Imbalance is yet another matter. It is often caused by pushing too hard to attain an extended position . . . one you cannot maintain. Chances are, if you're overly ambitious in doing the postures . . . you're the same way in "real life": always overextending yourself to no avail. So this routine will keep you from throwing yourself off balance.

In some cases, years of blocked or censored anger and fear lie locked inside our joints, muscles, and tissue—just like the rusty hinges on a forgotten door. Yoga will *physically* help to oil those squeaky *mental and emotional* joints, so that the door can open and close again at will.

There must be hundreds of variations on this theme, reminiscent of a Chinese puzzle or a Rubik's Cube. The fact is, each person is unique in the way the pieces fit together. Are you beginning to get the picture? The moral of the story is: *there is a significant correspondence between yoga and life.* The strengths and weaknesses we discover there translate themselves into our personalities and everyday circumstances.

In some cases, years of blocked or censored anger and fear lie locked inside our joints, muscles, and tissue—just like the rusty hinges on a forgotten door.

Come One and All

The beauty of this method is that anyone can do it, regardless of age, sex, or physical condition. That sets it apart from other fitness programs. Can you imagine, for instance, the average fifty-year-old man or woman hopping up and down incessantly or doing thirty-two leg-rises to rock music? Let's be realistic!

Calisthenics are not even a cinch for teenagers, so why should they be the jumping-off point for others less fit? It's like diving into the deep end before learning how to swim! We often have a tendency to act first and ask questions later—so it's not surprising that a number of us are caught huffing and puffing through some frenetic activity only to wonder, after all that effort, why we're still in such bad shape!

Without a fundamental understanding of the body—no matter what your goal is—you're going to come up short. First you have to know your own limitations so that you can work within them. But it doesn't pay off in reverse: by first exceeding your limits, and then trying to catch up. This puts you at a decided disadvantage. It's far more effective to build yourself to peak condition with a gradual approach. *Then* you can take on the rough stuff. The bonus is that, after a few months of yoga, most people are well able to hold their own in any exercise routine.

Robin Williams and Greta Garbo

Many professional athletes, dancers, actors, and actresses, who have conditioned their bodies through years of consistent effort, still come to this method for refinements they cannot obtain elsewhere. They don't view it as the shallow end, but as an end in itself. Many celebrities, including Greta Garbo, Yehudi Menuhin, Shirley MacLaine, Cary Grant, Gloria Swanson, Robin Williams, Tommy Tune, Juliet Prowse, Quincy Jones, Candice Bergen, and Louis Malle, have practiced yoga for separate reasons and goals as varied as the professions they represent.

The Rams and the Lakers

As a sports fan, I've often thought that certain physical culturists and sports figures could profit immeasurably from a regular dose of Hatha Yoga, and indeed many do. Members of the Los Angeles Rams and the Lakers have been known to practice this routine as a means of improving their games. As a concerned citizen, I cannot fail to notice a few flaky politicians (I'm sure you can name one or two) who need help gathering all their marbles together in one basket. Perhaps it could improve *their* performance as well. . . .

My Mom

I've seen my own mother—who suffers from an arthritic knee and could hardly walk—practice this method. That's right . . . at the age of sixty-eight, my sweet, dear, Rock of Gibraltar mother (who had never done anything physical in her life except: "I used to swim, darling, when I was a girl") started Hatha Yoga!

Not only did she start—she came to class every day without

Below: *My Rock of Gibraltar mom. She's got spirit!*

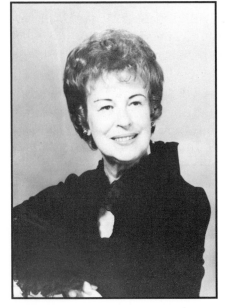

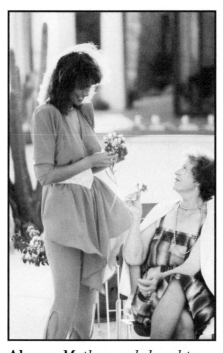

Above: *Mother and daughter—still close after all these years.*

fail. She'd drive her car forty-five minutes on the freeway to get there and forty-five minutes back just to do an hour and a half of yoga. But there she would be, with a smiling face, day in and day out—holding onto the wall at times for balance. There she was, in with all the younger students who could do all the postures better than she. . . . But boy, oh boy, she didn't give up—and she'd come out of a session just glowing.

Before long, she could walk much better. The swelling went down; the pain was relieved, and she wasn't suffering. Not only that! She looked as though she'd just had a face-lift. Only better. Lines were smoothed away, she had vibrant color without makeup, and clear, clear eyes.

I used to get a big lump in my throat watching her. I'd look behind me when we were in class together, see her smiling and struggling away, and damned if it didn't make me love her even more. I think she's really something. She's putting us all to shame. She's got real spirit!

A Small Price to Pay

Based on my personal experience and observations, I can't help but be especially enthusiastic about the possibilities this routine offers to people of all physical conditions. It's a common denominator that cuts through the boundaries of the physical culturists, and into the mainstream of Everyman. I'm not saying that it's the answer to every problem in the world, but, from what I've witnessed, it sure puts a dent in some rather common complaints like arthritis, bad backs, stiff necks, tension headaches, and high blood pressure—to name but a few.

I've seen a lot of women and men with health problems improve themselves through this method—people with steel pins in their joints, plates in their knees, legs twisted and malformed from injury. I've seen young girls who were so emaciated that their knees stuck out bigger than their thighs and their shoulders collapsed over their sunken chests—and in a year of practice they managed to transform themselves into beauties with shapely legs, filled-out flesh, and pretty faces, with shining hair and the glow of health. They do their yoga every day. It's a small price to pay. . . . What's yours?

Fundamentals

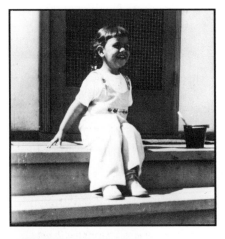

Above: *Me and my back porch, circa 1944, loose as a goose and on my way to flexible beauty.*

When we come into this world as babies, we're unafraid and loose as a goose. We can suck on our toes and fall all over the place with no problem. But later, in reaction to a myriad of physical and mental threats, our muscles stiffen up. They become so knotted up and intractable that sometimes they can even pull the whole spine out of whack. Since the spine houses and protects the power line to the entire nervous system, and since the central nervous system governs *all* the organs of the body—*including* the skeletal structure—this can make for big trouble. It's no wonder, then, that the flexibility of the spine is the cornerstone of all Hatha Yoga.

Flexibility and Health

Most animals stretch their spines instinctively upon awakening. But the human animal seems strangely negligent about taking care of the very backbone of his existence. The flexibility of the spine depends on regular manipulation (stretching and compressing) of the vertebrae to stimulate circulation and also to decalcify any deposits that might interfere with spinal mobility. Which is just a fancy way of saying that the improved flexibility you get from this method is a wonderful safeguard against the ravages of old age—arthritis, rheumatism, gout, and countless other maladies.

The Flexible Beauty

Flexibility has never been high on the list of priorities for women seeking beauty . . . probably because they don't know how important it is.

We are told that we can burn off fat. Although in a sense that's true, certain kinds of muscle pumping will only *firm existing fat into a hard mass*—solidifying all the bumps and bulges, almost as if preserving them in stone! First you have to get rid of these imperfections before you can tighten . . . otherwise the little devils get the impression you're inviting them in to stay for good!

Flexibility, beside being an unrivaled aid to good posture, also lengthens the muscles, giving your limbs a longer, leaner look that is most desirable. This sleek appearance is achieved by stretching your body, thereby releasing the pockets of tension that store the toxins. I marvel that so-called fitness experts seldom mention this.

A Chiropractic View of the Spine

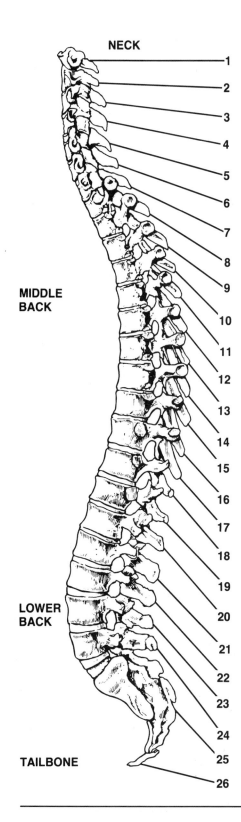

NECK
1
2
3
4
5
6
7
8
9
10

MIDDLE BACK
11
12
13
14
15
16
17
18
19

LOWER BACK
20
21
22
23
24

TAILBONE
25
26

	Area Supplied by Nerves	Possible Results of Nerve Impingement
	All tissues, glands, and organs are supplied with life energy by each spinal nerve.	Partial list of conditions and symptoms that may possibly result when there is an absence of life in the nerves
1	Blood supply to head, pituitary gland, scalp, face bones, brain itself, inner and middle ear, sympathetic nervous system	Headaches, nervousness, insomnia, head colds, high blood pressure, migraine headaches, mental breakdowns, chronic tiredness, dizziness or vertigo
2	Eyes, optic nerve, auditory nerve, sinuses, mastoid bones, tongue, forehead	Sinus trouble, allergies, crossed eyes, deafness, eye trouble, earache, fainting spells
3	Cheeks, outer ear, face bones, teeth, trifacial nerve	Neuralgia, neuritis, acne, eczema
4	Nose, lips, mouth, eustachian tube	Hay fever, rose fever, etc., catarrh, hard of hearing, adenoids
5	Vocal cords, neck glands, pharynx	Laryngitis, hoarseness, sore throat and other throat conditions
6	Neck muscles, shoulders, tonsils	Stiff neck, pain in upper arm, tonsillitis, whooping cough, croup
7	Thyroid gland, bursa in the shoulders, the elbows	Bursitis, colds, thyroid conditions, goiter
8	Forearms, wrists, hands, fingers, esophagus, trachea	Asthma, cough, difficult breathing, shortness of breath, pain in forearms
9	Coronary arteries, heart (including its valves and covering)	Functional heart conditions, certain chest pains
10	Lungs, bronchial tubes, pleura, breast, nipples	Bronchitis, pleurisy, pneumonia, congestion, influenza, grippe
11	Gall bladder, common duct	Gall bladder conditions, jaundice
12	Liver, solar plexus, blood	Liver conditions, low blood pressure, anemia, poor circulation, arthritis
13	Stomach	Nervous stomach, indigestion, heartburn, dyspepsia, etc.
14	Pancreas, islet of Langerhans, duodenum	Diabetes, ulcers, gastritis
15	Spleen, diaphragm	Stomach troubles, hiccoughs
16	Adrenal gland	Allergies, hives
17	Kidneys	Kidney troubles, hardening of the arteries, chronic tiredness
18	Kidneys, ureters	Auto-intoxication, skin conditions including acne, eczema, boils, etc.
19	Small intestines, Fallopian tubes, lymph circulation	Rheumatism, gas pains, certain types of sterility
20	Large intestines or colon, inguinal rings	Constipation, colitis, dysentery, diarrhea, hernias
21	Appendix, abdomen, upper leg, cecum	Appendicitis, cramps, difficult breathing, acidosis, varicose veins
22	Bladder, knee, sex organs including ovaries or testicles	Bladder troubles, many knee pains
23	Prostate glands, muscles of the sciatic nerve	Sciatica, lumbago, urination troubles, backaches
24	Lower legs, ankles, feet, toes, arches	Poor leg circulation, swollen ankles, weak ankles and arches, cold feet, weakness in the legs, leg cramps
25	Hip bones, buttocks	Sacroiliac condition, spinal curvatures
26	Rectum, anus	Hemorrhoids or piles, pain at end of spine while sitting

Right: *Stretching out in a dance routine from Broadway musical* Woman of the Year.

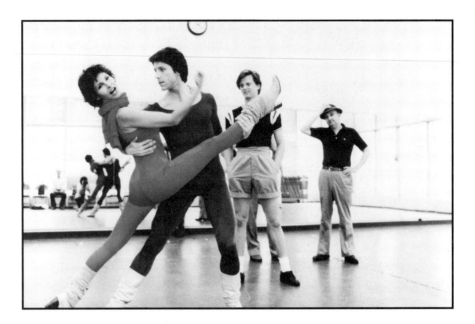

Below: *Strength is a very intoxicating, yet much misunderstood quality. With Ringo Starr in* The Magic Christian, *I seem to have the upper hand.*

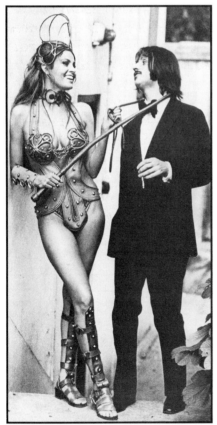

Can it be that they have not yet correlated premature aging of the tissues and cellulite with both mental and physical tension? It's elementary, my dear Watson, elementary.

This method of increasing flexibility while building strength reduces fat and cellulite by squeezing, wringing, and twisting the unevenness out of your skin as though by *self-massage*. The result is a smooth, unlumpy appearance free of those unsightly bulges.

Not bad for a low-priority item . . . perhaps it's time you moved flexibility closer to the top of your list. End of commercial.

Real Strength

Strength is a very intoxicating yet much misunderstood quality, and like beauty it is prone to oversimplification and stereotype. Which may be why so many men and women cultivate superficial strength to excess. Yoga doesn't build strength indiscriminately; it does so steadily, in relation to your need. The emphasis is on symmetry and harmony, not on bulk. Strength does not enjoy any precedence over other qualities here, as it does in other methods.

The ability to balance strength with flexibility is essential; otherwise, strength can become a liability. What good is a muscle man if he has no agility? Even with all his strength he's still a sitting duck. Remember the parable of the oak and the reed, in which the oak was struck down while the seemingly fragile reed survived the storm, because it was flexible in the wind? For that reason some weight lifters alternate between the gym and yoga to balance out their musculature and gain flexibility.

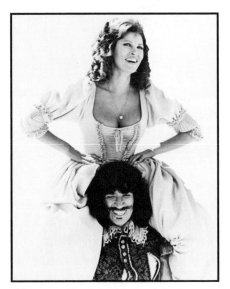

Above: *Trying to find balance on the shoulders of Frank Finlay in* The Three Musketeers.

In this method, muscular strength is seen as the principle of support. Your muscle structure internally *holds* your spine in place, lending support to your entire system and giving your limbs the ability to push and pull during movement or activity. In weight lifting or aerobics, you lift and lower your limbs or weights again and again in repetition. In this method, you assume a given position and *hold/support* your body weight *without moving* for ever-increasing periods of time. It's called staying power. This way, you work to build strength using only your body weight, rather than outside objects.

Finding Balance

Balance has always been one of the most sought-after qualities in the world. But, amid the chaos of the twentieth century, it becomes increasingly important to equalize the extremes and find inner stability. We've become more and more like acrobats walking a tightrope, with our sense of equilibrium our only means of survival. The frustration most of us experience trying to right the wrongs and correct the imbalances in our own lives, or even in society, is often overwhelming, and we begin thrashing around in desperation hoping to find a net.

Balance is inherent in each of us—if we know *where* to look. Often we don't see it because we search for it *outside of ourselves,* in others—for example, in our choice of partners. But when push comes to shove, we're left with only one solution: to find this center of balance *inside ourselves.*

That's where Hatha Yoga comes in. You may notice that all the poses in this routine are perfectly balanced. It's no coincidence therefore that as you perform them and achieve physical balance you'll also achieve *mental and emotional equilibrium,* thus killing two birds with one stone.

And who knows? If we can strive for and achieve balance on a personal level, we will perhaps be able to effect a significant change in the society in which we live.

Plunging In

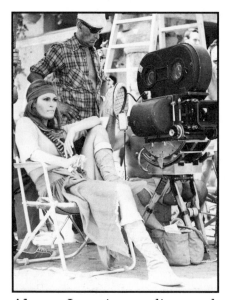

Above: *Learning my lines and lounging on the furniture. On location for* 100 Rifles *with Burt Reynolds and Jim Brown.*

This book represents a learning process. Like anything new, the techniques must be mastered before you can enjoy their full benefits. I found it to be a lot like memorizing lines from a script. Only after learning them can I play my part and the scene well.

The Learning Process

Learning yoga is no different. You can't "take off" until you get all those postures under your belt. The first order of business is to *give yourself time to absorb these new impulses* into your system.

Spencer Tracy once said his only rule for acting was: "Learn your lines and don't bump into the furniture." Everybody thought he was kidding, because it sounded so easy. Just try it sometime, and you'll see he was right. Learning is the hard part. And it takes time. So here's the bottom line. . . .

When?

The best times for practice are early morning—*before* breakfast—and early evening—*before* dinner. Always exercise on an empty stomach or allow at least one hour after a light meal or three to four hours after a main meal. If you are hungry before practice, try a cup of tea, milk, or fruit juice—that should do it.

The thing to remember is that in the morning your body will be slightly stiffer from the night's sleep, but this session will be very efficient in preparing you for the rest of the day and getting you ready for action. In the evening, your body will move more freely—your joints will be more limber, your muscles more flexible—and it's a great way to relieve yourself of any stress, fatigue, or tension you've accumulated during the day.

How Much Time?

Whatever your preference—mornings or evenings—make sure to set aside a little more than an hour, *every day*—a special time for yourself far away from distractions and interruptions.

"Impossible!" you say? Why don't you just try? Start by convincing yourself—and those around you—that this *is* the most important moment of your day. You'll be surprised to find how easily one can slip an extra hour into a 24-hour day! Remember, "Time is elastic." If Einstein said it, you better believe it!

The point is: better to do a little every day than to do a lot from time to time!

However, for those days when Einstein is proven wrong, when a little more than an hour seems like eternity, you'll find in the chapter entitled "Adapting the Method" three shorter routines: the Half-Series (a sequence of 40 to 45 minutes), the Mini-Series (a 25- to 30-minute set), and the Micro-Series (a quick session of 10 to 15 minutes). Once you know the entire basic program, they will still provide you with the essentials. The point is: better to do a little every day than to do a lot from time to time!

Commitment

Oh, brother, I can almost hear the moans and groans from here. At first, I didn't want to add anything to my already breakneck schedule either. I thought I'd rather "kill" myself once or twice a week and be done with it, than toil and sweat every day.

But the ever-present threat was there. I had to keep my "body beautiful" in shape for compulsory photographs, personal appearances, and those figure shots in my movies. It's my job. Sure, I'm interested in the metaphysical virtues, peace of mind, etc. But a piece of cake—cheesecake, to be exact—was the more urgent need that drove me at the time.

The rest came later—the nuances, the realizations. In fact, they crept in almost without notice. But what brought me through the door and into everyday practice—make no mistake about it— was my vanity. If you're a little vain, too, then get yourself in gear and make the time and the commitment.

Where?

You'll need an area large enough for you to stretch, equipped with a full-length mirror—to check and monitor your postures— and, if possible, a carpet. A pad, a mat, a folded blanket, or even a large towel laid down on the floor will also do.

The room should be warm—*never,* I repeat, *never* exercise in a cold or air-conditioned place: your muscles will be stiff and you could injure yourself. I bought myself a portable electric heater— it sure helps those early winter mornings! (I even use a vaporizer when the air is too dry.)

Note: Athletes and dancers are forever warming up and protecting themselves from chills, so I've often wondered why health clubs have air conditioning *blowing directly* on the bodies of people who are working out—it's purely and simply dangerous!

What to Wear

Any kind of loose-fitting and light clothing that allows you complete freedom of movement will do. I wear leotards. For guys,

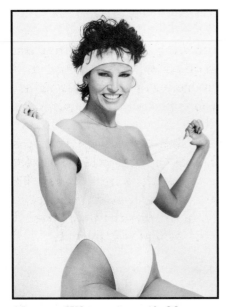

Above: *What to wear? Choose something unforgiving and strive to live up to it.*

What's terrific about this method is the immediate feedback you enjoy, which is very encouraging for the beginner. There's nothing like instant success!

fitted briefs or shorts are perfect. Just forget tights and hose, and remove your watch, eyeglasses or jewelry. Beware of those outfits that look great but restrict your breathing in any way—that includes your skin—and circulation. The lesser, the better.

All right, in the dead of winter you may add tights and leg warmers, but heating the room is better. Your skin—or epidermis—is the largest breathing organism on your body: don't suffocate it!

I know, you were counting on a bit of camouflage to hide those dimpled thighs, but tell yourself this is the last time you're going to look this way. Those bumps and bulges aren't *you*, anyway—they're just excess baggage that you're about to unload!

How?

Each posture leads very precisely into the next—adding to or balancing out the one before—by progressively warming, stretching, and toning all the muscles, joints, ligaments, and tendons of your body. Therefore, it is very important that they be performed in the *exact order* indicated in the book, following the step-by-step instructions exactly.

Note: Before you start the postures, here are two important things to remember as you proceed through the method.

1. Follow the step-by-step instructions under each photo carefully for specific information on *which side* (left or right) to start each posture. The photos demonstrate the action *only*, but do not necessarily reflect which side to start on.

2. REPEAT means to do the entire posture again *on both sides.*

I also recommend that you read through the entire posture section thoroughly before starting to do the poses. It will make it easier for you.

The Method to the Madness

Each of the postures is performed *twice*. The first set is designed to "program" your body and get it used to the positions. The second set reinforces those signals and takes you further. Let's say the first set is to break the ice, the second set makes friends. Once you're warmed up and more flexible, you can get better acquainted and make progress! So make more of an effort in the second set—that's the one that helps you improve faster. What's terrific about this method is the immediate feedback you enjoy, which is very encouraging for the beginner. There's nothing like instant success!

Follow Through

The second day goes better than the first; the third day continues the momentum you started. Every succeeding day you'll add more small victories to your list, so please don't miss the second or the third day, or you'll start to forfeit all you've gained. It's too soon to start cutting corners.

The speed and regularity of your triumphs will no doubt boost your confidence, because this method always responds to consistent effort. However, it's a two-way street: you can't cheat. The gains for a beginner are like those of no other sport, exercise, or physical discipline, but can vanish as easily as they appear. If you're off and on in your practice, the results will show it.

At Home

When you start out learning at home, you may not get all the way through the postures the first time. This is perfectly natural if you are working on your own. Try doing just four or five poses in succession; then add a few more each day as you go. Always go back over the ones you already know to begin each session, and stick to the order shown. Then proceed to learn some new ones. After you've tackled all twenty-eight poses separately, start to do two sets of each position or cycle. Little by little does it every time.

Dry Periods

Once you've mastered the process—which will take you from thirty to sixty days, depending on your fitness level and perseverance—it's like money in the bank. After your initial investment, it starts to earn interest. Even if circumstances outside your control conspire to make you miss practice, your body's memory bank will hold the postures in safekeeping, ready to be reclaimed.

I've been amazed to find that after certain intervals, even the most difficult poses were still imprinted indelibly on my reflexes. They just needed a little dusting off.

A Movable Feast

When I first started this routine I was really gung ho and doing it every day in California. But after thirty days, I had to go on location in Paris to shoot a movie called *L'Animal,* with French star Jean-Paul Belmondo. The prospect of turning my back on all my hard-earned gains was unthinkable! So I decided I'd have to do it on my own. I started out with great trepidation in my hotel room, in the heart of Paris, and—mon Dieu!—found to my amazement that yoga is a movable feast.

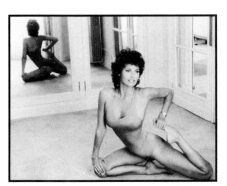

Above: *Have mat, will travel. Yoga is a movable feast. From Paris to Timbuktu, I stay in training.*

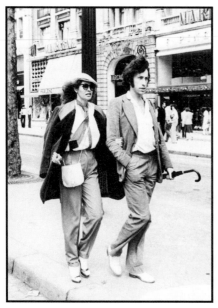

Above: *Strolling the Champs-Elysées in 1977 with* un type français *who later became my husband.*

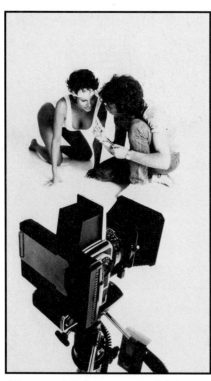

Above: *André, me, and his Hasselblad, on the job together.*

I kept myself in shape for my figure-revealing costumes in the film, and it gave me enough energy after a day's shooting to flirt shamelessly with *un type français*—one particular Frenchman who later became my husband! André thought the whole thing was a hoot! He'd come by to pick me up at my hotel room and invariably find me caught in the midst of an extraordinary pose—whereupon he'd sink down into an overstuffed chair and watch agog. "Boy, oh boy, you American girls are really something!" was all he ever said.

Have Mat, Will Travel

I've done this routine in Mexico during photo sessions, in Las Vegas during my nightclub act, on Broadway while doing *Woman of the Year,* in the Caribbean on vacation, in Montana shooting *Walks Far Woman,* in London, Rome, and Tokyo. Wherever I go, it goes. What's that you say? You don't have the discipline. Don't let that stop you. . . . Just *do* it! You're the only person you can depend on. You never can tell what'll happen when you're out there on your own. You can forget your toothbrush, but don't forget to pack your yoga.

Nobody's Perfect

In yoga, there is no comparison or competition, except with yourself, and no standard of perfection, except your own. No two people are the same, so no two postures will look identical. How "perfectly" you do the postures doesn't matter—just do *the best you can,* on any given day, at your own rhythm and pace, and you will progress faster and better than you ever thought.

Don't be discouraged, though, if—while growing more confident—you experience a temporary setback or if your improvements seem to slow down. Yoga is a progressive method. Your body will still be going through important changes, but without your being *aware* of it. So, don't force or strain; arm yourself with patience, determination, and faith, and within a few days, you'll be relaxed and smiling again.

Inspiration

If the photographs in this book inspire you—as I hope they will—that's great! But please stop short of being intimidated by them. Be assured that each shot is the result of a lot of blood, sweat, and tears. They may look easy in their final finished form—calmly executed without a hint of strain. But over the years I've fallen down, cried, stomped my feet, cursed, walked away, and started again. The point is, I'm still doing it. Why? Because it's worth it!

Shall we begin?

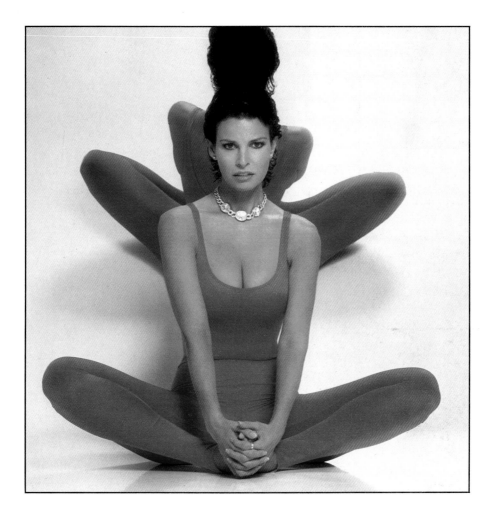

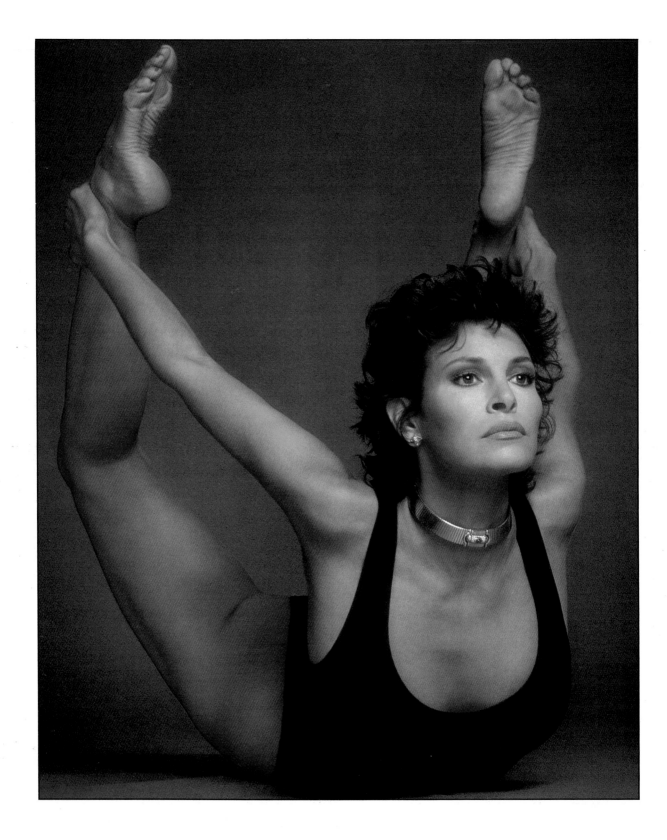

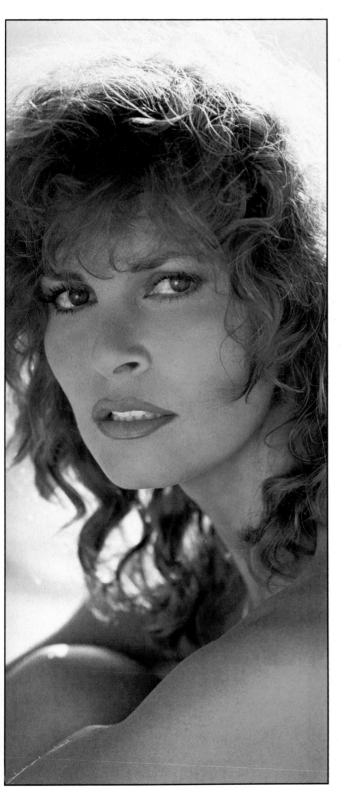

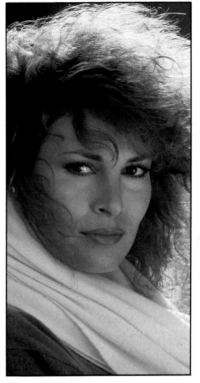

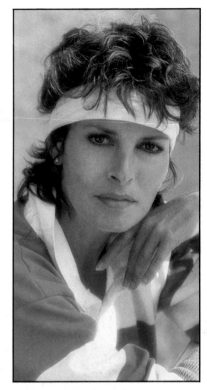

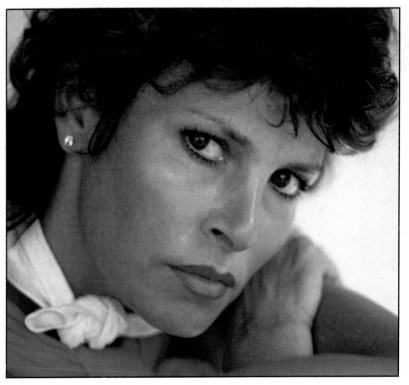

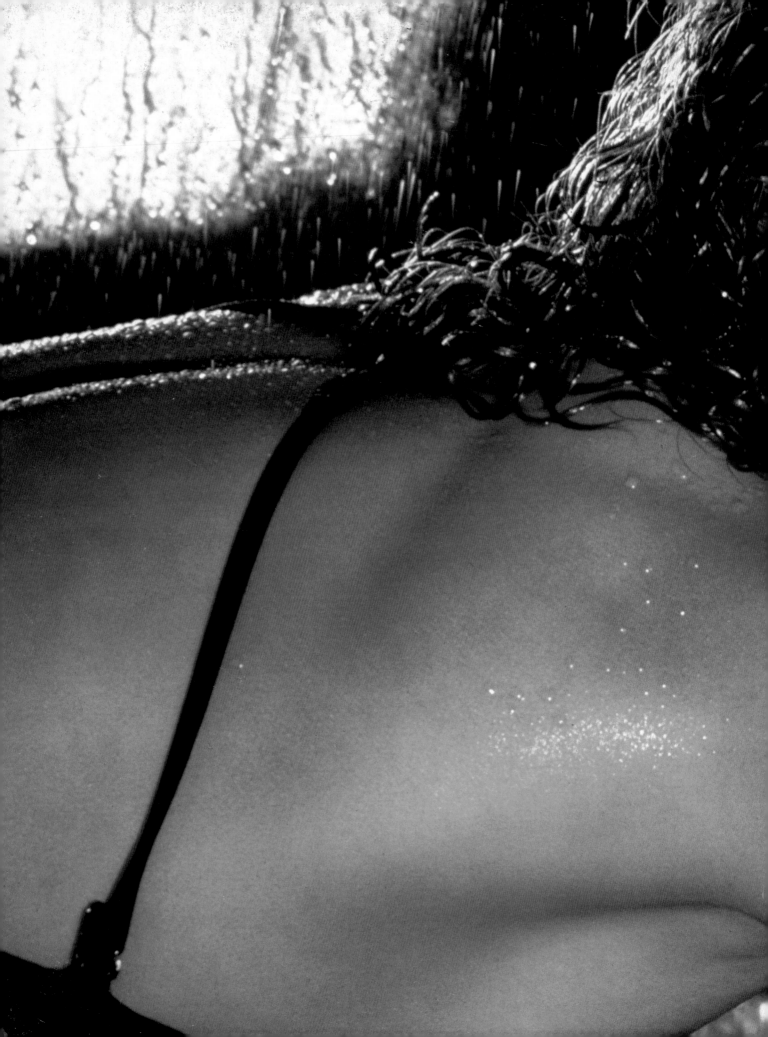

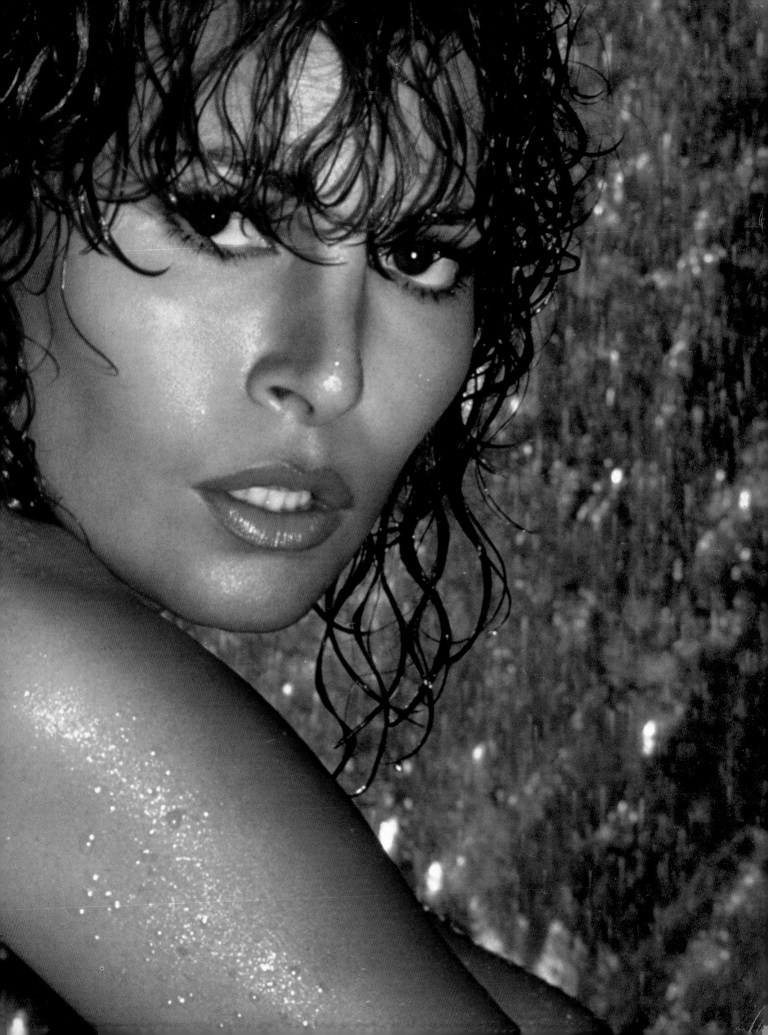

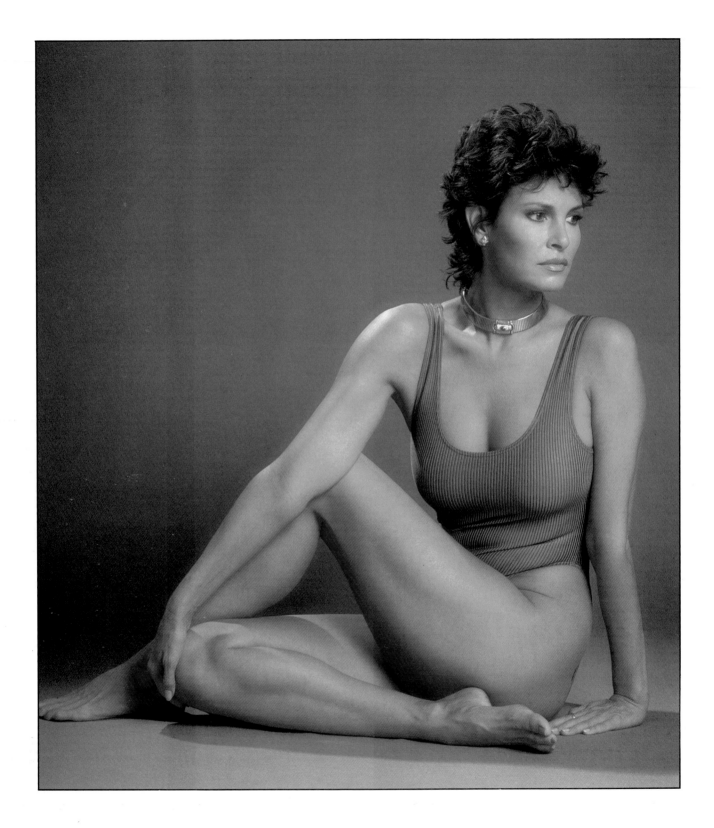

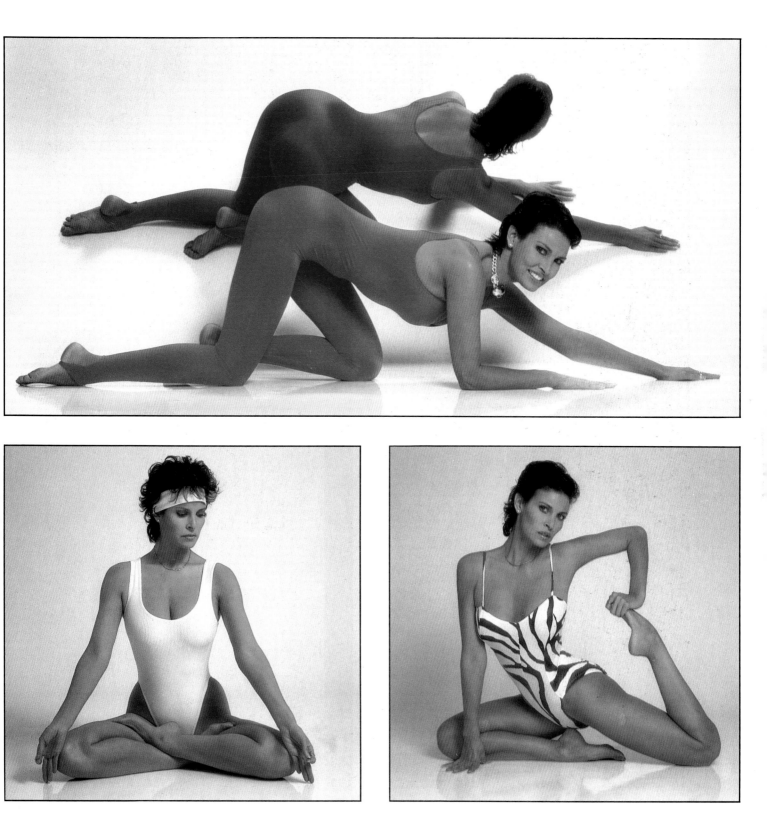

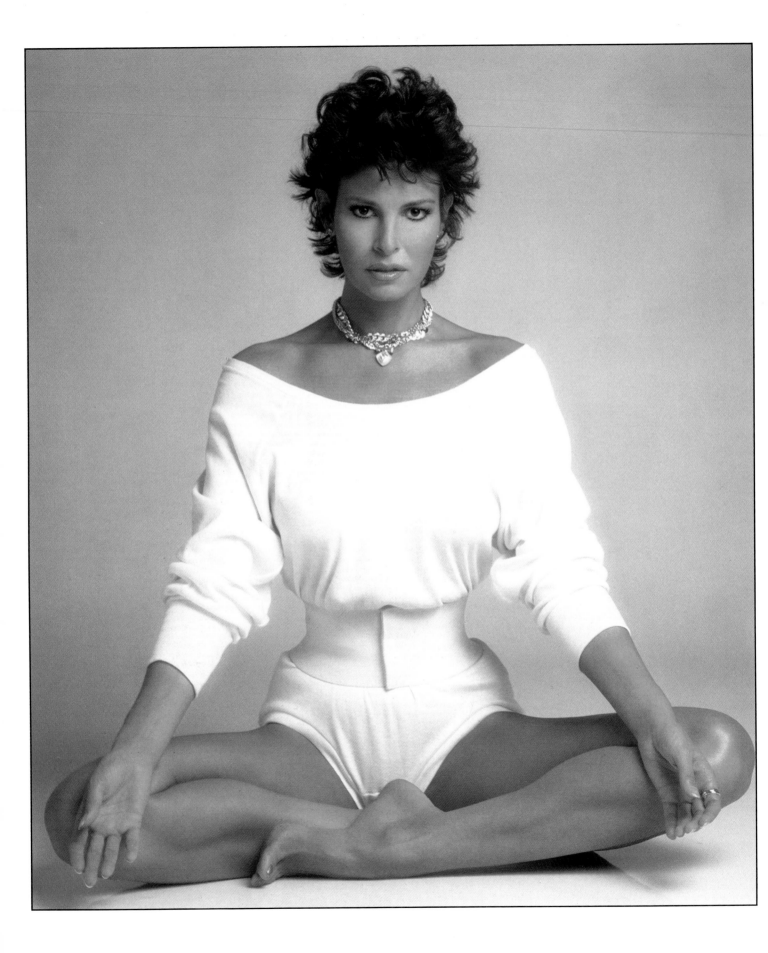

The Postures

The Fabulous Five

If you practice this method regularly, not only will you gain physical strength, flexibility, balance, and energy but you will also benefit from the following mental qualities:

1. Concentration
2. Balance/Equilibrium
3. Determination
4. Patience
5. Faith/Confidence

Those are the tools you need to pursue your own ideals and goals in life. This method is a road map with lots of options, so you must chart your own course and make your own discoveries. Your destination is a matter of choice—but it's the journey there that counts.

BREATHING

Deep Breathing Number 1

I regarded breathing like someone I loved dearly and couldn't live without, taking it for granted, neglecting it . . . and then, wondering what happened when it was gone.

Breathing is the *only* beginning. It's the beginning of life . . . and it's the beginning of this learning process. But, you may ask, "What is there to learn about breathing?" After all, we trust that we'll inhale and exhale automatically and involuntarily every second of our lives. Is there such a thing as breathing wrong? It almost seems like a contradiction in terms.

I've found that unconsciously I used to commit every sin imaginable against good breathing, from holding my breath when I was nervous to hyperventilating during strenuous activity. Needless to say, I was often at a disadvantage, because my body was in a state of almost perpetual panic. I regarded breathing like someone I loved dearly and couldn't live without, taking it for granted, neglecting it . . . and then, wondering what happened when it was gone.

Because I used to take breathing for granted, it's hardly surprising that the breathing exercises described here held absolutely no interest for me. At the same time, they were very difficult to perform in the early stages. For weeks, I "faked it," so I could get on to the "good stuff." I just did the arm and head movements regularly, without giving the breathing itself much thought, and—lo and behold—in spite of myself I experienced a breakthrough. Just when I least expected it! Now, I wouldn't dream of starting a day, much less this routine, without it.

Air is your most essential food. To inhale is to drink in and feed yourself on the spirit of life. Do so with relish. To exhale is to release the miseries and pressures that attack your serenity. Do so gladly. Eat and drink all the air you want: it's nonfattening.

Benefits

- Increases the capacity of the lungs (most people use only a fraction of their lung potential).
- Releases stress and tension.
- Calms the mind and emotions.

Note: This is not meditation. It is a no-nonsense preparation for physical activity.

Deep Breathing

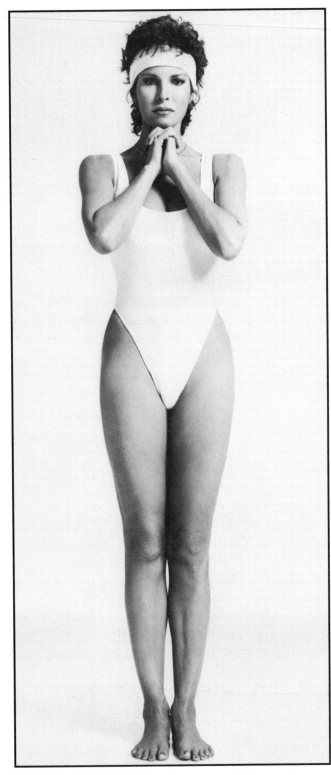

1. Stand up straight, facing a mirror. Put your hands together under your chin, with your elbows almost touching.

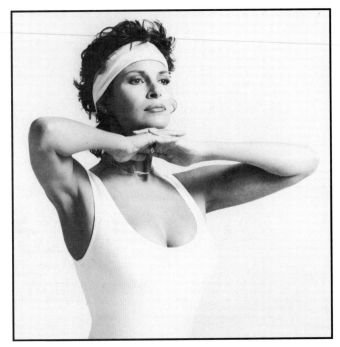

2. Now, inhale slowly for 6 counts through your nose (mouth closed), *feeling the air in the back of the throat.* At the same time, lift your arms to the side.

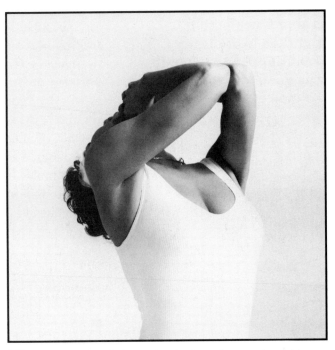

5. As your head drops back, the elbows should come together slowly. Try to make your forearms and face into a straight line.

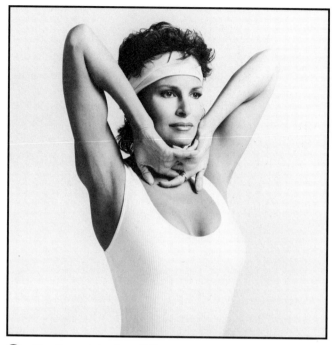

3. Continue inhaling, lifting your elbows until they are as high as they will go. Press down with your chin against your hands. You *must* feel the breath vibrate off of the vocal cords in your throat.

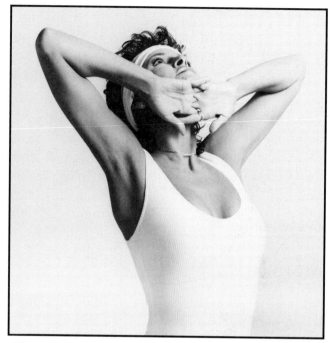

4. At this point, let your head drop back and your mouth open gently. Exhale for 6 counts slowly through your mouth.

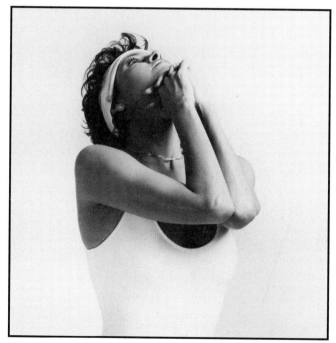

6. Bring your head slowly forward. Next, begin another cycle by inhaling through the back of your throat for 6 counts. Once again, you will get a vibrating sensation on your vocal cords.

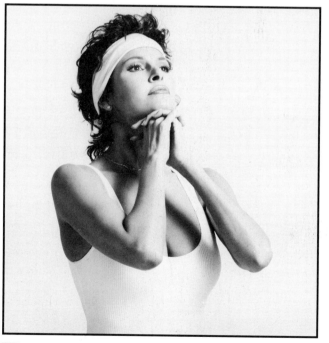

7. As your head comes forward, your elbows should open up as before, and you should follow along with step 2. Do a full cycle of 10 breaths, inhaling and exhaling each time. Rest briefly with your arms at your sides and then REPEAT.

Deep Breathing

Extra Help

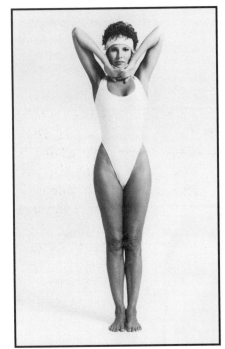

Above: *This is the correct stance for the Deep Breathing cycle. However, if you have trouble with dropping your head back, bend your knees slightly (keeping them together).*

1. **Standing.** Most other programs let you stand with feet and legs apart, but not this one. It looks deceptively simple but it's more work to hold your balance and your body erect with your feet and legs together. Don't let yourself have duck feet or ballet turnout.

2. **Inhaling Through the Throat.** The concept and feeling of air brought through the nose and *throat* is no doubt something new to you. It doesn't take much time to get used to it, though. Remember to keep your mouth closed when inhaling—this insures that the air automatically comes through the nose. As it does, try to feel the sensation of the air vibrating in the back of your throat. If you make whirring, snoring, or gurgling noises, you're on the right track.

3. **Exhaling.** When you exhale, do so through slightly opened lips. Don't be surprised if the sound of the air changes as you push it back through your throat and out your mouth. Try to do so with control and don't let it escape all at once. Direct it going *out,* as well as coming *in,* against the back of the throat. Going out, it usually has more of an "aah" sound. That's a good sign. It means you're doing it correctly, but you're just a little rusty or congested. If you sound like you have a case of terminal consumption, don't worry. You'll soon be purring away nicely.

4. **Elbows.** Some people have difficulty getting their elbows all the way up—by the ears—in the first inhale motion. Others find that they resist coming together at the top during the exhale. It all conspires to make you feel like a real klutz. Don't despair. As a beginner, your flexibility will improve with practice. Be patient.

5. **Head.** If you can't get much play in the forward and backward movements of your head, don't be discouraged. If it's any consolation, everyone has days when shoulders and neck are stiff—they are the seat of a lot of tension. This is your opportunity to breathe through and work it out.

6. **Wrists.** Try not to let your arms break at the wrists during these movements, except when your elbows move up past your chin. Otherwise keep your forearms in a straight line throughout.

7. Dizziness. Because breathing deeply is new to you, you may feel slightly lightheaded. Don't be afraid, you won't fall. The antidote is to *keep your eyes open* and resist the urge to close them. As long as you stand correctly as described in step 1, this posture will hold you firmly so that you can breathe deeply. But keep your eyes open, and your dizziness will subside.

8. Stamina. What seems like an easy exercise at first may have you gasping and sputtering like a broken-down jalopy. Can you really be that out of shape? The answer is yes. As a beginner, when I was only halfway through, I was ready to drop. But it's quite normal to experience difficulty, both inhaling and exhaling *fully,* for the first time. How difficult it is reveals just how much you need it. So keep going. Your stamina will improve and your breath will run smoothly before long.

What seems like an easy exercise at first may have you gasping and sputtering like a broken-down jalopy. Can you really be that out of shape? The answer is yes.

Words of Encouragement

I can't tell you what a boon deep breathing is to the rest of these postures. It sets you up great for the whole series. Once you've got the breathing down, you've got it made. Breathing is your strongest ally when you're called to action. Funny, isn't it, that such a small thing could affect us so much? Yet it does. It sets up a body rhythm that you'll be able to follow right through the posture and out into life.

Isn't it good to know that you can work to your own tempo, instead of to rock music?

STRETCHING

The Reed/Hands to Feet

Shaking up your body like a bottle of prefab salad dressing is better than nothing, but definitely not as good as making your own from scratch.

Most warm-up exercises I've experienced involve bouncing. Bounce, two, three, four . . . generally to the relentless beat of rock music. While this may be stimulating, it stops short of doing the job. Shaking up your body like a bottle of prefab salad dressing is better than nothing, but definitely not as good as making your own from scratch. So bouncy warm-ups are never as beneficial as an *even* and *uninterrupted* flow of blood and energy.

But if stretching isn't bouncing, what is it? A stretch is not a bounce, or a push or a jerk or anything violent, but rather the *holding* of a position—*without forcing*—at its most extreme point. The body itself, in its own wisdom, then releases and allows you to pass through that point of tension/resistance.

The secret is to *put yourself on hold* . . . to find the position and stay there. When done smoothly and quietly, a stretch reveals signs of tension, stiffness—or, conversely, *over*flexibility—to your body's ear. Listen to it. Let the intelligence of your body work for you. Respect what it says about how far to go and how fast. Before long you will have created that "inner dialogue" we spoke of. Now you can see why we don't need music, we're making our own.

Benefits

Reed Pose (steps 1–10)

- Stimulates and stretches the upper body in three directions.
- Limbers the spine and strengthens the muscles of the shoulders, back, and abdomen.
- Firms and slims the waistline.
- Tones and stimulates the abdominal organs such as the stomach, kidneys, and liver.
- Improves blood circulation and builds energy and vitality.

Hands to Feet (steps 11–20)

- Adds flexibility and strength to the spine.
- Limbers the hamstrings, improves the flexibility of the tendons and ligaments of the legs.
- Tightens the muscles of the back, stomach, and legs.
- Tones the nervous system and the abdominal organs, helping digestion.
- Increases blood circulation to the legs, head, and facial tissues.

The Reed

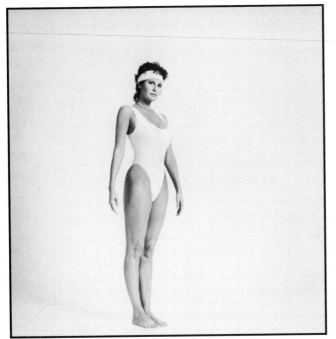

1. Stand up straight, tighten your buttocks and abdomen, and lift your rib cage. Do not let your upper torso sag. This is the beginning stance for all the standing postures.

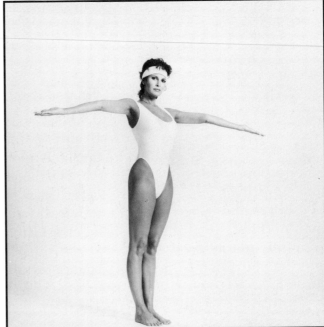

2. Begin to raise your arms to the side slowly, in a straight line. Keep your elbows locked.

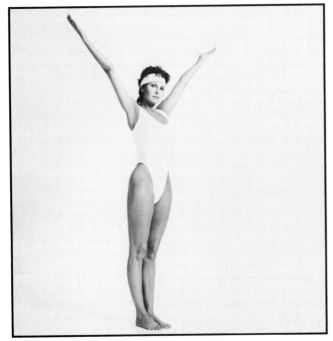

3. Continue to raise your arms and lift your upper torso higher as you go. Keep your shoulders relaxed.

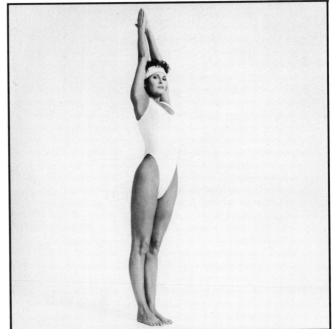

4. Place your hands together, interlocking your thumbs. Your fingertips should point and reach for the sky. Get your arms in as close to your ears as possible.

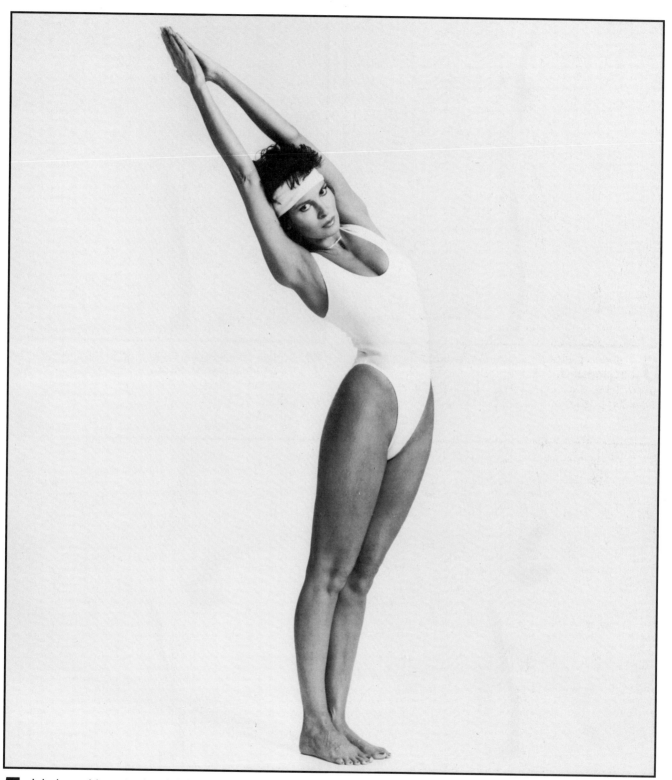

5. Inhale and lean to the right. Exhale when you reach resistance; then continue to breathe normally. Feel the stretch on the left side of your body, right through the fingertips. Try not to let your chin drop against your chest and hold this position for 10 counts. Come back slowly to the center, inhale and lean to the left. Stay in your best stretch for another 10 counts, breathing normally. Do not repeat, go straight to the next step.

The Reed

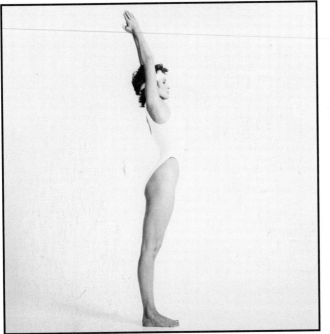

6. Come back again slowly to the center position and inhale deeply.

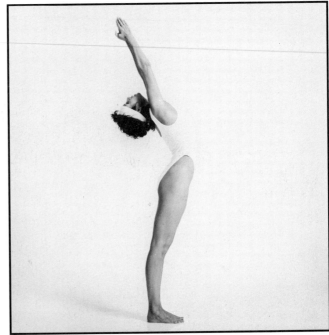

7. Exhale and drop your head gently to the back, as far as it will go.

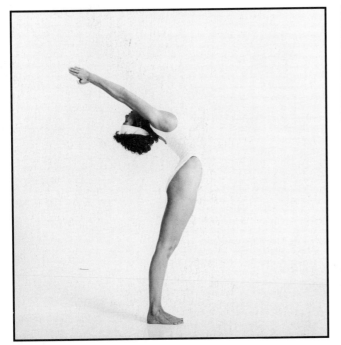

8. Now inhale again and start to reach backward with your arms and begin your arch, breathing normally as you go.

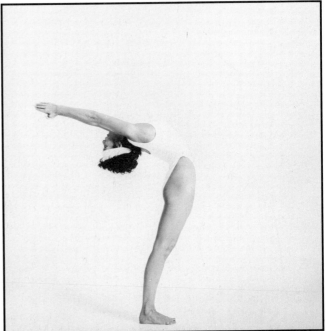

9. Allow your back to release and arch backward still farther, feeling the stretch along the front of your body. Press your hips forward, concentrate on exhaling to release any tension, and keep your weight on your heels.

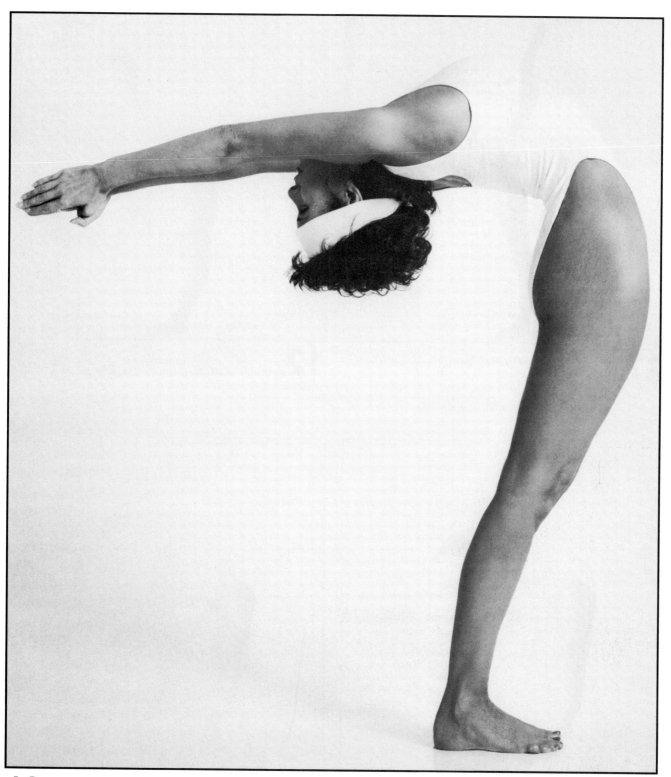

10. When you are arched to your farthest comfortable point, hold the position for 10 counts, breathing normally. Keep reaching backward with your arms and pushing forward with your hips. Bend your knees slightly if you have to.

Hands to Feet

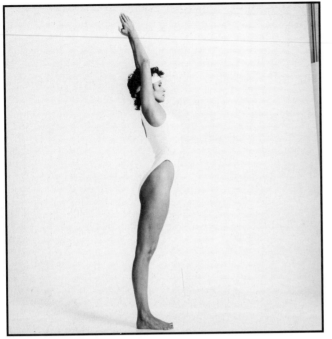

11. Come back up *very slowly,* allowing your head to clear for a moment. Then, inhale.

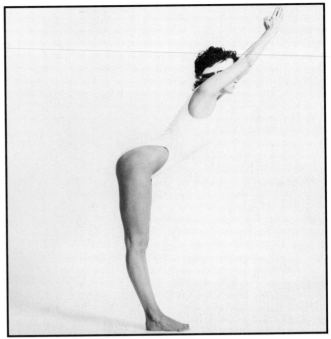

12. Now start to bend your body forward in a straight line from your hips. Exhale smoothly as you go.

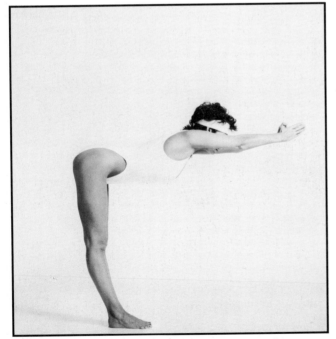

13. Start reaching forward, feeling the pull down the back of your legs. Make sure your legs are straight, your knees locked and your feet together.

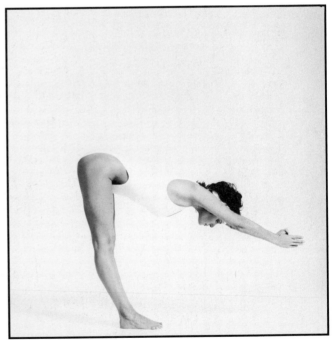

14. Continue to keep your torso in a straight line all the way down. You may feel your weight shift slightly to the center of your feet.

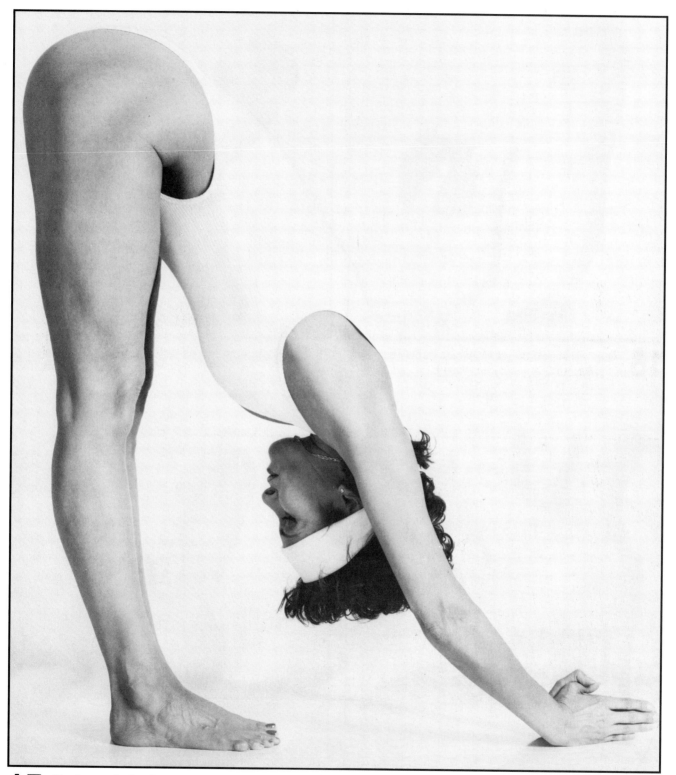

15. Try to touch the floor in front of you without bending your legs. See how far you can go. Keep remembering to breathe normally.

Hands to Feet

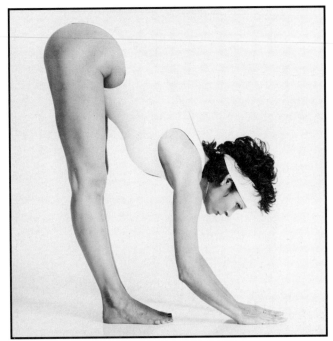

16. Now start bending your elbows, allowing gravity to pull your body weight closer to your thighs. Let your hands slip back along the floor toward your feet.

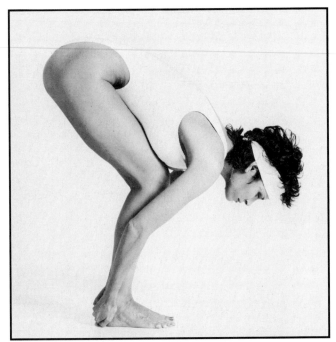

17. Bend your knees and take hold of your ankles. The proper grip is fingers wrapped backward around the heels and thumbs on the bottom touching the floor.

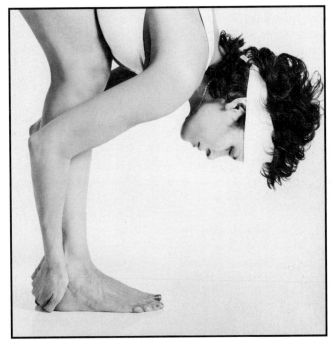

18. Pull with the strength in your arms against the heels, as you slowly straighten your legs. Concentrate on exhalation when you meet points of resistance.

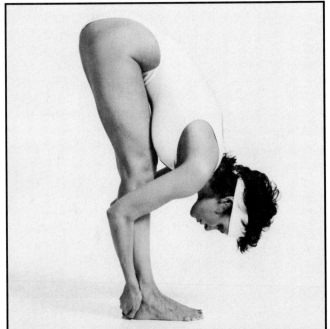

19. As you straighten your legs, keep your elbows glued to the sides of your calves and your chest touching your thighs.

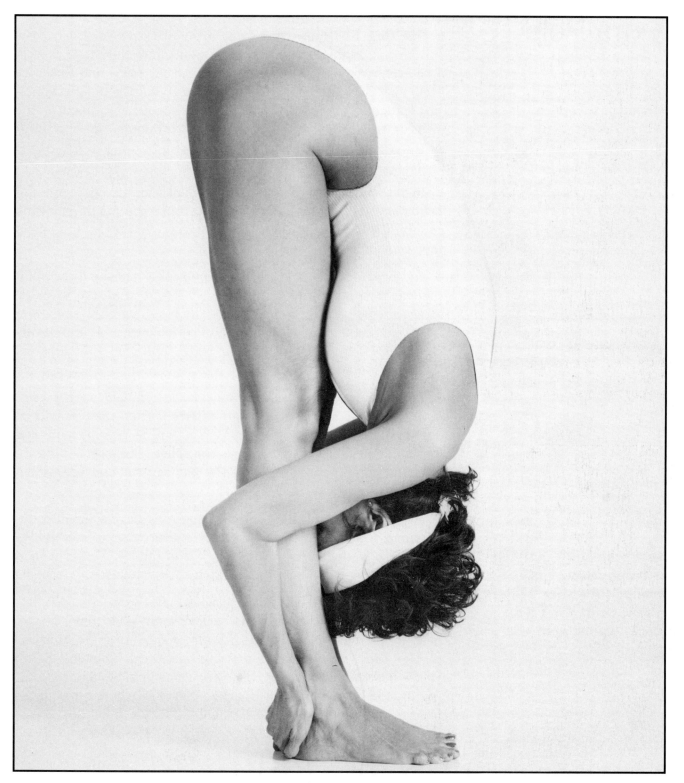

20. Finally, drop your head to your legs if you can, your face touching the shins. When you get to your best position, even if you close your body into the legs, hold for 10 counts. After the count, release your grip on the heels and rise slowly, the same way you went down, keeping your hands together and your arms extended in front of you. When you are back to center and upright, rest and REPEAT the entire cycle again.

The Reed/Hands to Feet

Extra Help

Just remember that fear is synonymous with tension—it's your enemy. Abandon it, don't let it work against you.

1. **Starting Position.** Once your arms are over your head, you will have a tendency to let your chin sink into the chest. Don't— if you tuck your hips under and stomach in, you'll find that your head and chin set perfectly straight on your shoulders, almost automatically. Also, think about keeping your chin about 3 to 6 inches away from your chest—it varies throughout the posture.

2. **Staying Power.** In calisthenics, you beat or pound away repetitiously at your points of resistance. In this method, the idea is to go to the most extreme point, which varies from day to day, and *hold there,* breathing, relaxing, sustaining the maximum effort calmly. It's the only way to fly and it gets results. So start using that principle now, on the Reed/Hands to Feet.

3. **Side Stretch.** Your hips should push the opposite direction to the way your arms are pointed. Don't try to go all the way over by sacrificing your correct position. The results are the same even if you can manage to stretch only a few inches: you'll still get the slimming effect. Don't twist your body, and keep your hips and shoulders square to the mirror.

4. **Uneven.** In this pose, when you stretch from left to right, you'll notice that one side is completely different from the other. Don't despair. This is absolutely normal. You will always be more flexible on one side, and stronger on the other. No body is perfectly even. As you practice, however, the gap in your unevenness will begin to close.

5. **Fear of Falling.** As a beginner, you may have some difficulty dropping your head back all the way and arching your body. But this phase passes, along with your fear of falling. Just remember that fear is synonymous with tension—it's your enemy. Abandon it, don't let it work against you.

6. **Back Bend.** First relax the back of your neck, then let your head drop. Trust yourself. Then *think of stretching the front part of your body,* as opposed to arching backward. This will help if you're frightened of falling. Use your arms to make an arc, pointing up and over at the wall behind you. Feel the stretch up the front of your thighs, and press your hips forward. It's this tension that will compensate for the backward pull. Also, *keep your weight on your heels and your eyes open.*

7. Stiffness. If you encounter a point of stiffness, persevere and breathe through. The small of the back is the favorite spot for all fears and doubts to rest. So just relax, don't tense up, follow the directions above, and have confidence. Nothing will happen to you.

8. Dizziness. Coming out of the back bend can make one a little woozy. So, come up slowly, allowing your circulation to equalize. Again, *keep your eyes open.* Until your stamina is built up you may feel weak, but resist the urge to drop your arms, and keep them aloft until you bend forward. Hold on, help is on the way.

9. Forward Bend. The main thing to remember is to bend forward from the tailbone. Even when you bend the knees to grip your heels, think of lifting your hips. The object is to gain flexibility in your hip joints.

10. Knees. Just bend your knees as much as is necessary, so you can place your hands on those heels. If you can't, keep trying, your time will come. Many yoga programs do not have this feature, so use it. If you're a beginner, it's a great way to build flexibility in the legs and hips without hurting yourself.

11. Coming Up. Coming out of the forward bend, don't drop your composure—the pose is not over yet. Lift yourself up slowly, arms over head, and when you're upright, drop them to the sides with control. Now you can rest. Sustained effort counts a lot in yoga. It builds strength and energy.

Words of Encouragement

When your head clears from this posture, you are going to be more awake than ever. Your body has been stimulated in every direction and the cobwebs in your mind will begin to disappear. Even on rough mornings, this is the one that gets me going. It's well worth the effort and something you'll come to enjoy.

Besides, the second set is easier than the first. By then, you'll be well on your way.

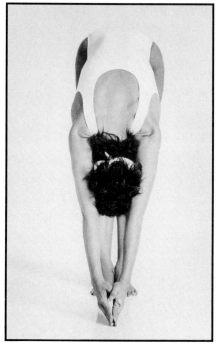

Above: *Keep your arms and head in this position as you come back up to center. Hold your composure until the end.*

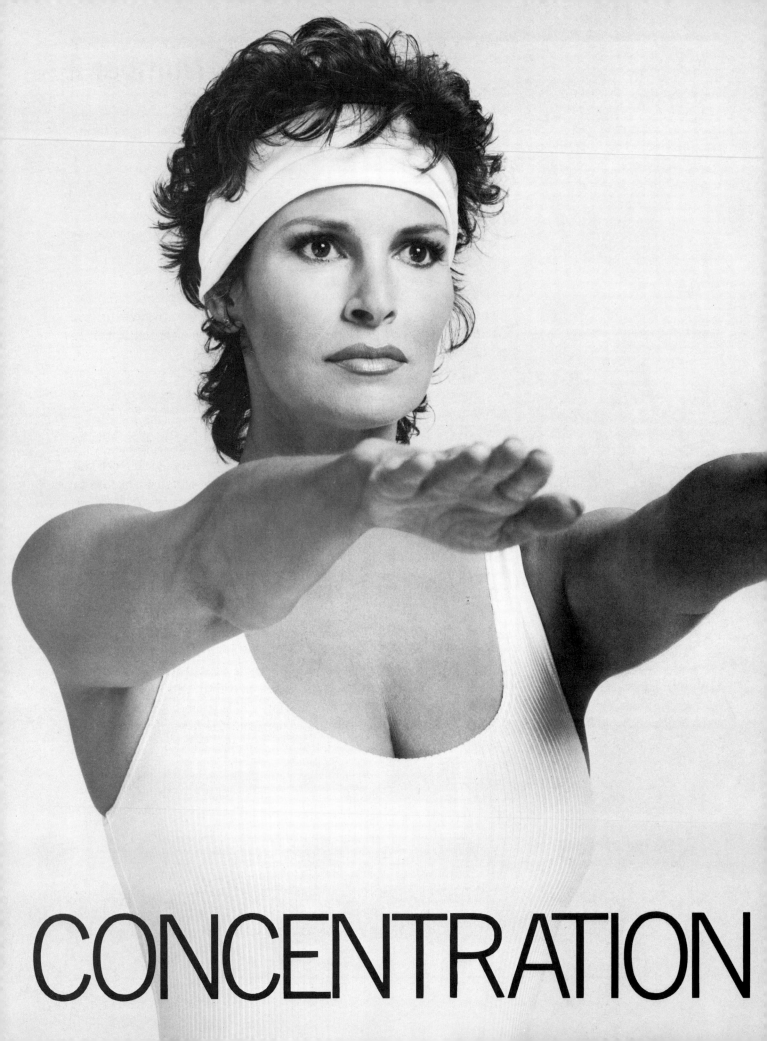

CONCENTRATION

The Chair Pose Number 3

This posture helps you to *concentrate,* which the dictionary defines as "to direct toward a common center or objective" or "to increase the strength of by removing foreign elements." Either way, I'd venture to say, it's a concept alien to most Americans. The truth is that many of us have lost the art of concentrating or focusing our energies on a given task for a sustained period of time. We give our attention only momentarily until something better comes along, conditioned—by the ubiquitous TV commercials—to having our thoughts constantly interrupted. Initially, we may have been annoyed, but, slowly and surely, we've become accustomed to it. No wonder that, at this point in our evolution as a high-tech society, we have an attention span of about 30 seconds! Look around you. People are skimming instead of reading, are unable to carry on a conversation because they don't listen or even wait for the answers to their questions. You've probably noticed how often you see two people talking at once!

The situation is bleak, but not hopeless. It's totally unnatural to have our minds bandied about like Ping-Pong balls, but it's up to us to reverse it. This method can help. The Chair Pose helps you to find your "center," fix it, and hold on to it as you move through the posture. It helps you to block out those "foreign elements" that prevent you from accomplishing the task at hand. None of this three-part pose is a snap (they don't even have the *appearance* of being easy). But they can be mastered more easily than you imagine. The key to it all is *concentration.*

Benefits

- Improves and strengthens the muscles of the legs, and helps them develop evenly, particularly the thighs and calves.
- Corrects minor deformities of the legs.
- Limbers and strengthens the hip and ankle joints.
- Provides flexibility and tones the upper arms, shoulders, and lower spine.
- Helps relieve spinal disorders such as slipped disc, lumbago, backaches, etc.

The Chair Pose

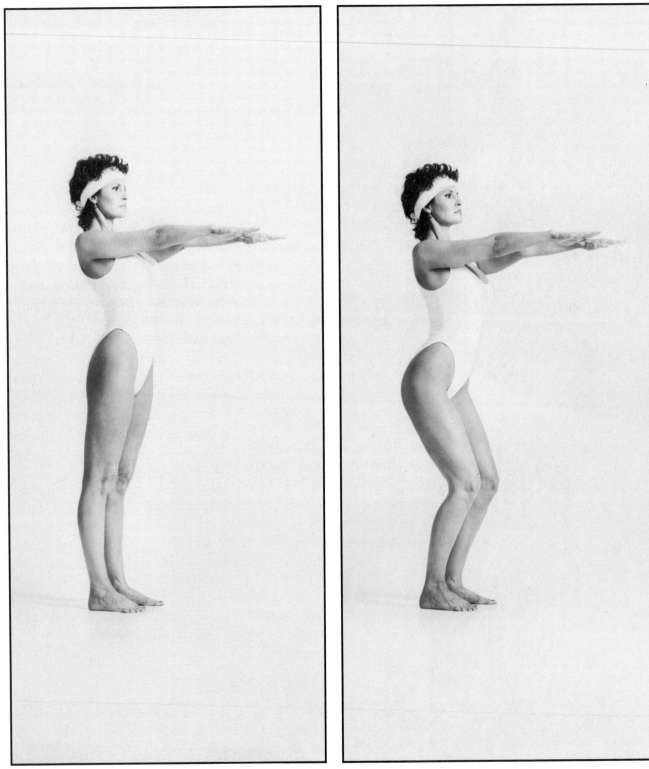

1. Stand up straight, arms extended firmly at shoulder level. *Fix your eyes on one spot* in front of you and don't move them throughout the posture. This will help your balance.

2. Bend your body at the knees and hips only, and begin to "sit down" on an invisible chair behind you. Stick your bottom out backward and keep your knees and feet 6 inches apart.

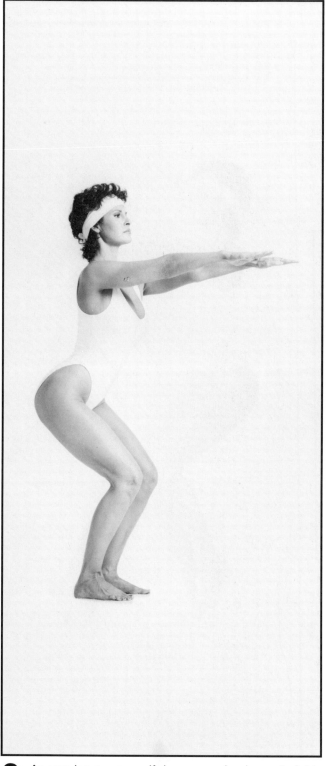

3. As you lower yourself, keep your back as straight as possible. Keep your weight on your heels. Feel yourself lean backward.

4. Try to get your thighs parallel to the floor and your back at a 90-degree angle. Use your back and thigh muscles as well as the abdominals to hold yourself in place for 10 seconds. Breathe normally.

The Chair Pose

Extra Help

Below: *In the third stage (steps 9–12) of the Chair Pose, your arms and thighs should be parallel to the floor and your back should be at a 90-degree angle.*

Below right: *If you have trouble with your balance, use your arms as levers to regain your center, while maintaining your* one-spot *gaze.*

1. Straight Back. The real killer here is trying to keep the back absolutely straight. Few people can do so, but keep this image in mind. It seems the farther down you go, the farther forward you lean. Keep your weight on your heels, even if you feel your toes lift slightly. And lean back against your imaginary chair. Work it, it's worth it.

2. Arms and Legs. Ideally, the thighs and arms should both be parallel to the floor. And that's not easy at first. Never mind. As long as you make your best effort you'll improve quickly. Remember to keep the knees 6 inches apart. Don't let them close together. And keep your arms and hands tight—they are important too.

3. On Your Toes. Don't be discouraged by the sight of this pose. It looks harder than it is. Lift up on your toes, just fix your gaze, press your instep forward and lean farther back. Stay there and concentrate on your breathing. If your legs shake a little, let them. It's a very good sign that things are happening.

4. Lower Yourself. When you sit on your heels in the last stage, lower yourself all the way down with control and composure. Don't drop down suddenly. Maintain balance and a straight back every inch of the way and go *slow*. It's better for you.

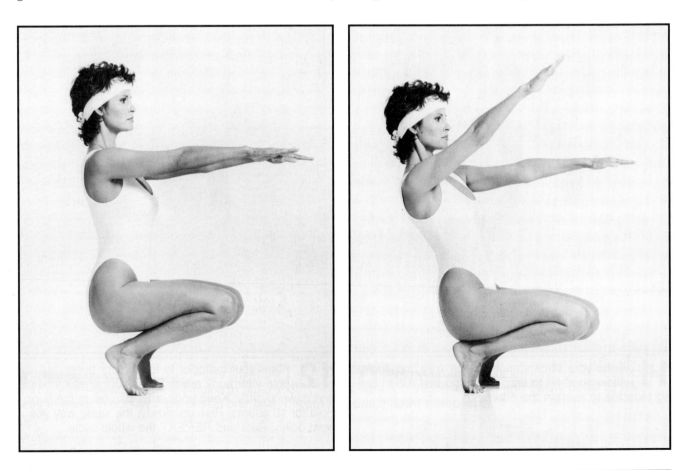

Words of Encouragement

The Chair Pose is quite difficult, but not impossible. Not by a long shot. In fact, for all its difficulty, it does remarkable things for the legs, even for those who practice it only moderately well. It develops tone and definition like nothing I've ever seen. So keep at it.

In addition, once you've mastered it, I think you'll regard it—as I do—as a turning point, a barrier broken down, a means of centering your concentration and focusing your energy. No matter how susceptible you are to distractions and discouragement, this posture will help release the hold of outer forces on you. It actually excludes the intrusions and makes it possible to pursue a single line of endeavor.

When you acquire the ability to execute this pose, you will find your own "center," making it possible to concentrate and direct yourself *totally* in any given situation. This posture is worth its weight in gold!

No matter how susceptible you are to distractions and discouragement, this posture will help release the hold of outer forces on you.

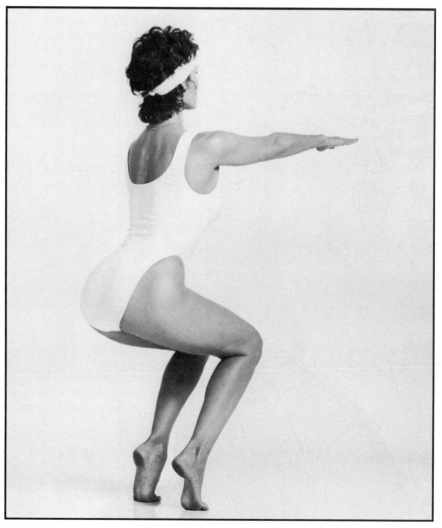

Right: *This pose looks harder than it is—I was surprised how quickly I got it. If your legs shake a little at first, let them. It's a good sign that things are happening.*

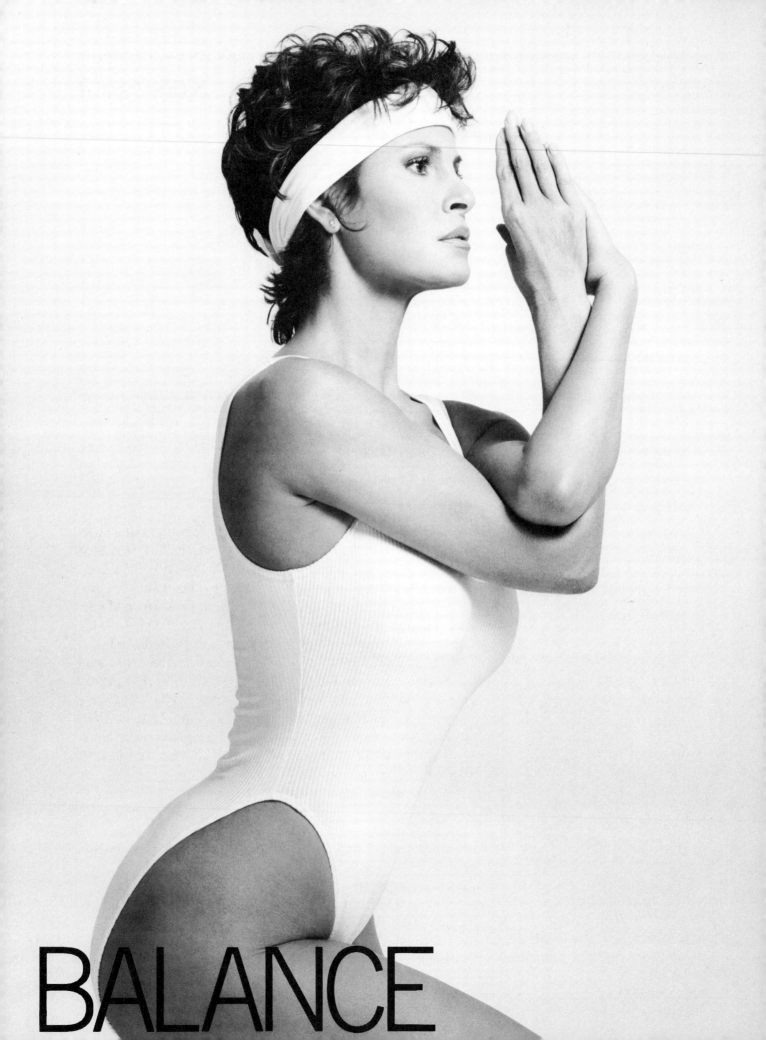

BALANCE

You will not be molding yourself into anyone else's image, but into your own distinct physical and mental identity.

Up to this point we've explored proper breathing, the importance of flexibility, and the need for concentration. Now it is time to combine all these elements together in the practice of *balance*. This is the first posture in the series that requires you to balance on one leg. This skill will enable you to work each leg independently, to strengthen it and make it more flexible, so that the health and agility of *both* sides of the body will be improved.

We'll start slowly, using two legs to balance on one. You may think of it as one leg standing and the other leg molding—shaping itself into the perfect complement for the other. You will not be molding yourself into anyone else's image, but into your own distinct physical and mental identity. With that prospect in mind, let's attack the balancing series and begin what is sometimes an awkward process with enthusiasm.

Benefits

- Strengthens and improves the flexibility of the leg muscles, especially the thighs and calves.
- Tones the upper back muscles.
- Works and limbers the shoulder, hip, knee, and ankle joints.
- Stimulates and tones abdominal muscles and organs.
- Increases blood circulation in the arms, legs, and extremities.
- Develops balance and concentration.

Eagle Pose

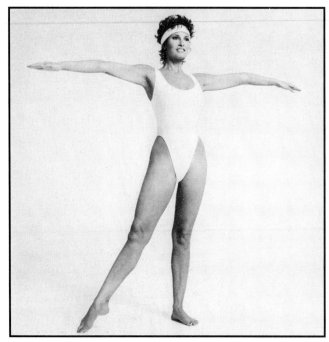

1. Stand up straight and open your arms to the side, at shoulder level. Point your right leg out to the side as well.

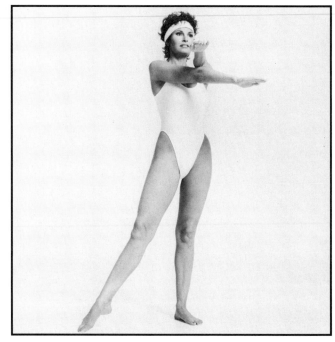

2. Now, fix your eyes on a spot ahead of you and cross your right arm under the left one.

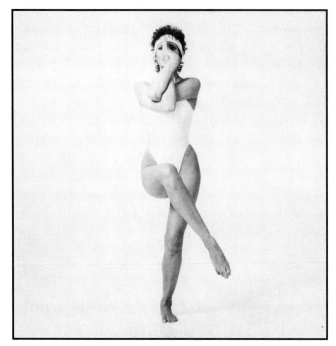

5. Once your arms are intertwined, sit down about 6 inches on your standing leg and begin to wrap your right leg over your left leg. The rule is: The right arm crosses *under,* while the right leg crosses *over.*

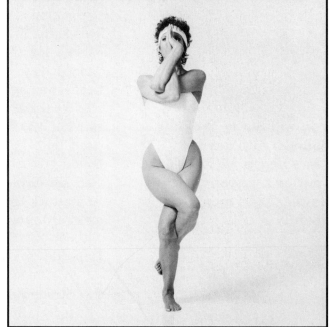

6. Continue to twist the right leg over, under, around and through the leg you are standing on and stare past your fingers at your fixed spot for balance. Adjust your hips so that they are even.

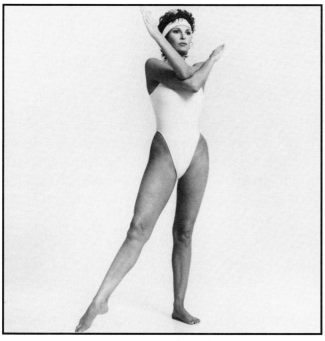

3. Bend your elbows, holding your gaze through the arms.

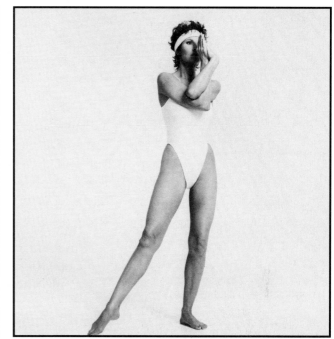

4. Wrap your arms around each other and join the palms together in front of your face. At the same time, begin to bend your standing leg slightly.

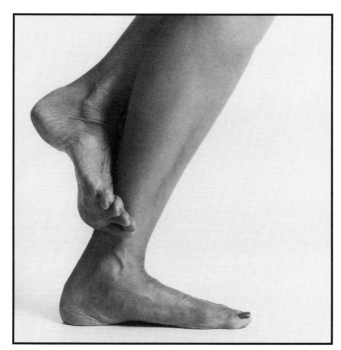

7. Your foot should hook around the opposite ankle, letting your toes peek out the other side.

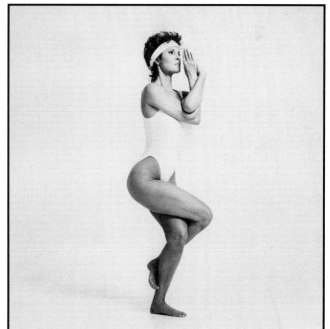

8. Once in the twisted position, pull your elbows down to your chest, settle onto your standing leg, and squeeze your legs together. Keep that back straight. Hold for 10 counts. Unwind arms and legs, rest. Do the other side. Then, REPEAT.

Eagle Pose

Extra Help

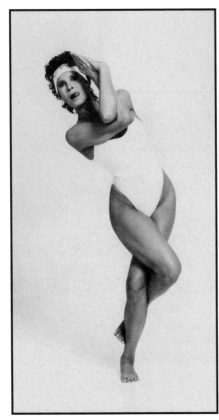

Above: *Ooops! Everybody has awkward moments—that's what keeps you on your toes. You have to concentrate to maintain your balance.*

Opposite: *Since balance is one of the most important benefits of this method, fix your gaze and concentrate on that spot. It's key to all the poses that require balance.*

1. Arms and Hands. Try using the momentum of swinging your arms together from the sides in order to wrap them around each other. If your palms and fingers don't touch, do the best you can. Hang in there—in a week or so it'll be much easier. Remember to pull your elbows down to the chest. This speeds the process.

2. Legs and Feet. The best policy for problems with the legs and feet in this pose is the slow wrap. Squat down on one leg and steady yourself, then lift your other leg *up, over, around and through.* Hold your best position, gradually the gap will close between the legs and your toes will come around. Remember, you're just starting!

3. Balance. For most people the device of fixing the gaze on one spot is enough to gain balance. If you have more trouble, sit farther down into the pose. But if your balance is extremely shaky, you may lean against a wall while adjusting your arms and legs; think nothing of it, it's better than falling over. Gradually rely less on the wall, as time goes on. This method is for everyone, it's not a performance or competition. It's what the body gains that counts.

4. Leg Squeeze. The best way to get optimum benefit from this pose is to "sit" well into it with a straight back and *squeeze your legs together.* It helps to get your hips even.

Words of Encouragement

This can actually be a quite beautiful pose when done correctly. Once again, it's a pose designed to mold your legs into great shape while you're twisting them. So sink into it willingly, with commitment.

This is your first single-leg balancing pose and will require your full concentration.

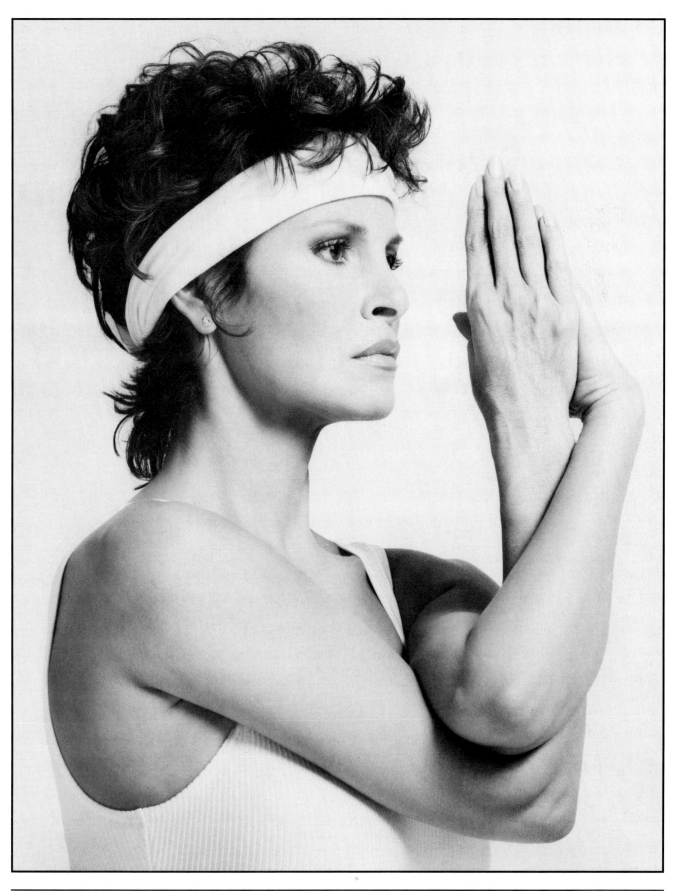

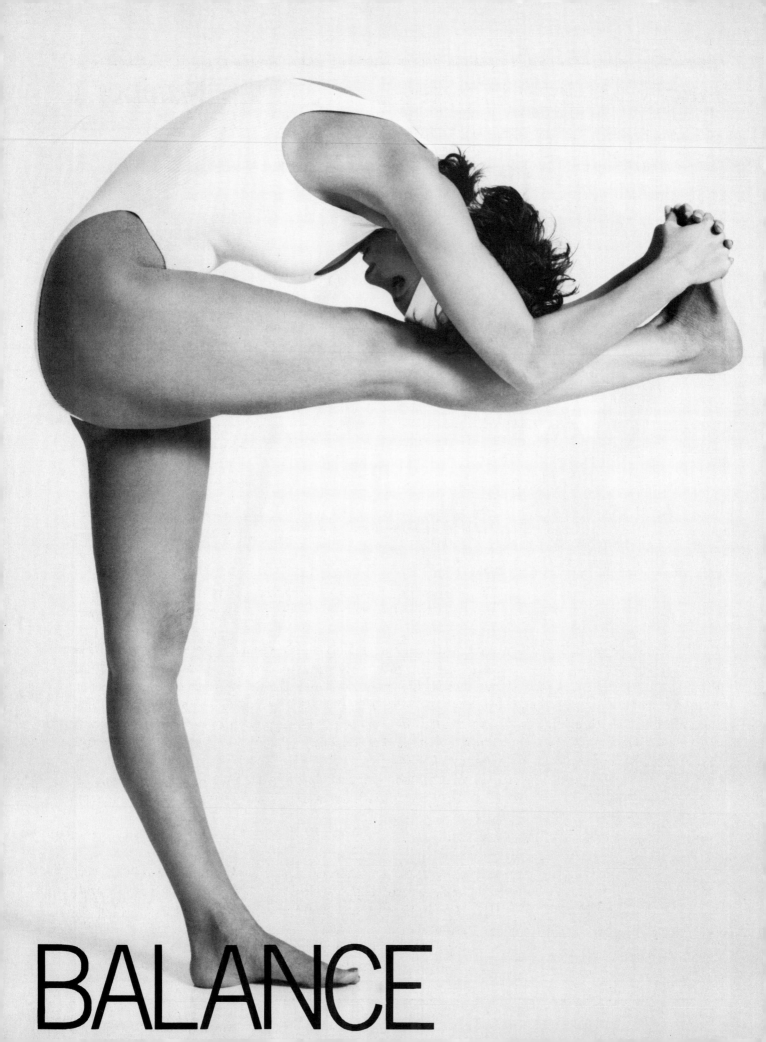

BALANCE

Standing Head to Knee Number 5

Within thirty days, despite my initial pessimism, I found myself doing this impossible pose! I've since discovered that the only thing in our way is doubt.

The first time I saw the following posture I was dumbstruck. The Standing Head to Knee seemed to defy gravity, and a voice inside me said, "Never . . . you'll never do it." I was deeply intimidated—and made an effort only to see what would happen. Within thirty days, despite my initial pessimism, I found myself doing this impossible pose! I've since discovered that the only thing in our way is doubt. We've got to stop judging and fearing and just start to *do*. What seems like a tough posture in the beginning will soon seem easy! When that happens, it builds your confidence like nothing else can.

Note: These balancing postures are invaluable and seldom included in other fitness programs. So take advantage of them here.

Benefits

- Strengthens and tones the muscles and ligaments of the back, abdomen, and legs, particularly the thighs and calves.
- Adds flexibility and stretches the hip joints and the sciatic nerves.
- Improves digestion and tones the liver, spleen, and kidneys.
- Promotes coordination, concentration, and balance.

Standing Head to Knee

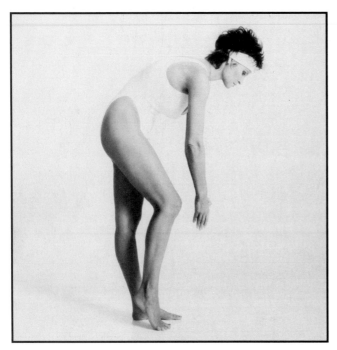

1. First, shift your weight onto your left leg, and prepare to pick up your right foot. Keep your standing leg *absolutely straight* from the beginning.

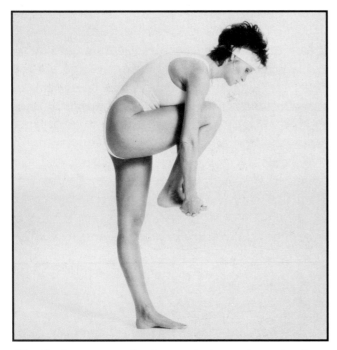

2. Find a spot on the floor or in front of you that is comfortable and set your eyes there. Now, take hold of your foot slowly and hold it there firmly for a moment.

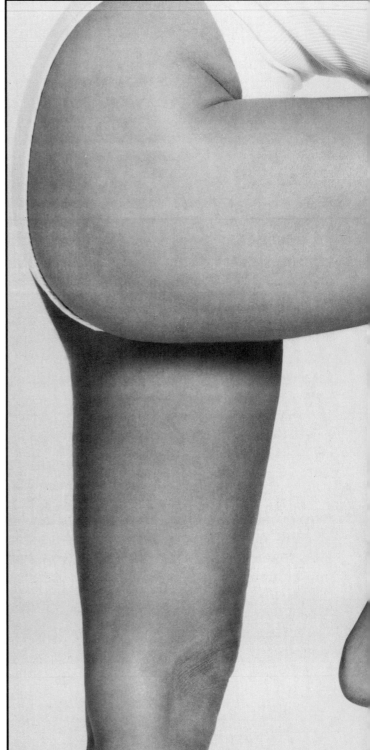

3. The grip on your foot should be fingers wrapped around the ball of the foot under the toes and the thumbs crossed over the top of them. Now, keeping your standing leg absolutely straight and locked, start to extend your other

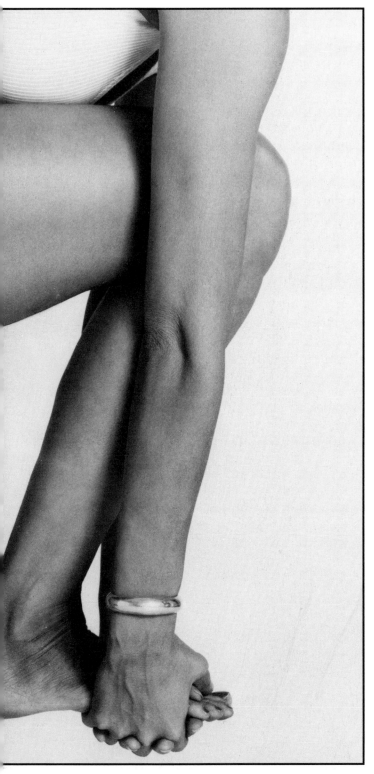

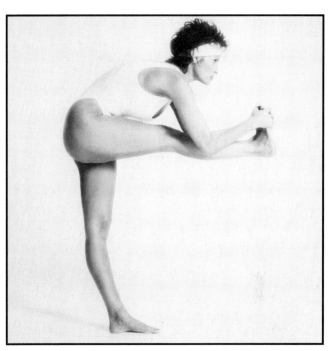

4. Stay in your best position, even if your leg is not straight, for 10 seconds. Breathe normally. If you have good balance, you can change your gaze to check your position in the mirror (beginners should not try this).

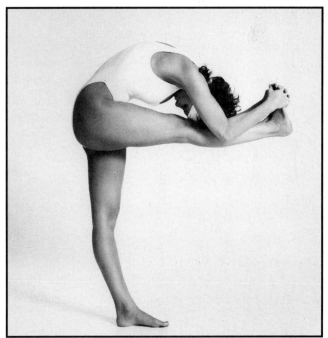

leg forward and up, pushing with your heel, while pulling back on your toes. Bend your elbows as you go, and keep them close to the side of the leg.

5. If you can, drop your head slowly to the knee. Keep pulling on your toes and press the heel forward. However, if you cannot straighten your leg completely, do not try this last step. Rest, do the other leg, and REPEAT.

Standing Head to Knee

Extra Help

Even if your leg feels overextended down the back, don't be scared. Don't tense up, try to relax into it.

1. **Foothold.** When you slip your foot into the stirrup of your hands, hold it *firmly*. Get a good steady grip because that may be all you can manage to do the first day. But that's good. Take everything one step at a time.

2. **Locked Leg.** My teacher, Bikram, always said that *keeping the knee locked is the most important thing* to do in this pose. So even if you don't get your leg out in front right away, concentrate on your standing leg. In this method, a straight leg is more than just straight—it must arch back behind the knee. To attain this, *relax and breathe,* allowing your joints to open up. Even if your leg feels overextended down the back, don't be scared. Don't tense up, try to relax into it.

3. **Pulling.** Once you can stand holding your foot steadily, slowly extend your leg forward and up. *The main thing here is to pull like mad against your toes, and push your heel forward simultaneously.* This will give you control and balance. *Keep pulling* even if you feel a tension in the back of the knee. It will take time for your sciatic nerve and lower spine to release.

4. **Eyes.** If you're having trouble holding your position and find yourself hopping around, or maybe even falling to the side, *remember to set your eyes on one spot* and don't move them for anything. This is your point of concentration, *watch it, breathe, and relax.*

5. **Head to Knee.** If, after all your efforts of pulling and pushing and holding, you still cannot straighten and lock your extended leg, do *not* attempt to drop your head to the knee. This is a no-no. You're not ready for it.

Words of Encouragement

There's no doubt that this pose is quite formidable at first, but you will be able to accomplish it if you can relax and concentrate.

For beginners, active relaxation will come easier if you realize that there's no reason to be scared. Nothing will break. What will happen, however, is that your joints will open, sending a fresh supply of oxygen and energy throughout your body. Success is just around the corner in this pose, if you keep on trying!

By the way, after the first few postures, your heartbeat will be relatively the same as if you were doing aerobics. But in yoga, it builds gradually, without a shock to the system. You may not be aware of it, but you are steadily building momentum and stamina. Take advantage of it. Be sure not to lollygag around between sets because the breathing rhythm which is established in the first set will help support you in the second.

Below: *These photographs illustrate spotting in the mirror (as in step 4), instead of on the floor. Once your balance is more steady, you may want to look straight ahead as you extend your leg forward.*

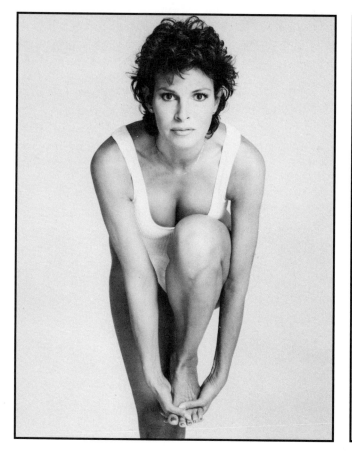
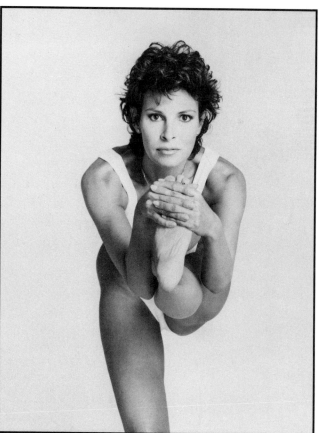

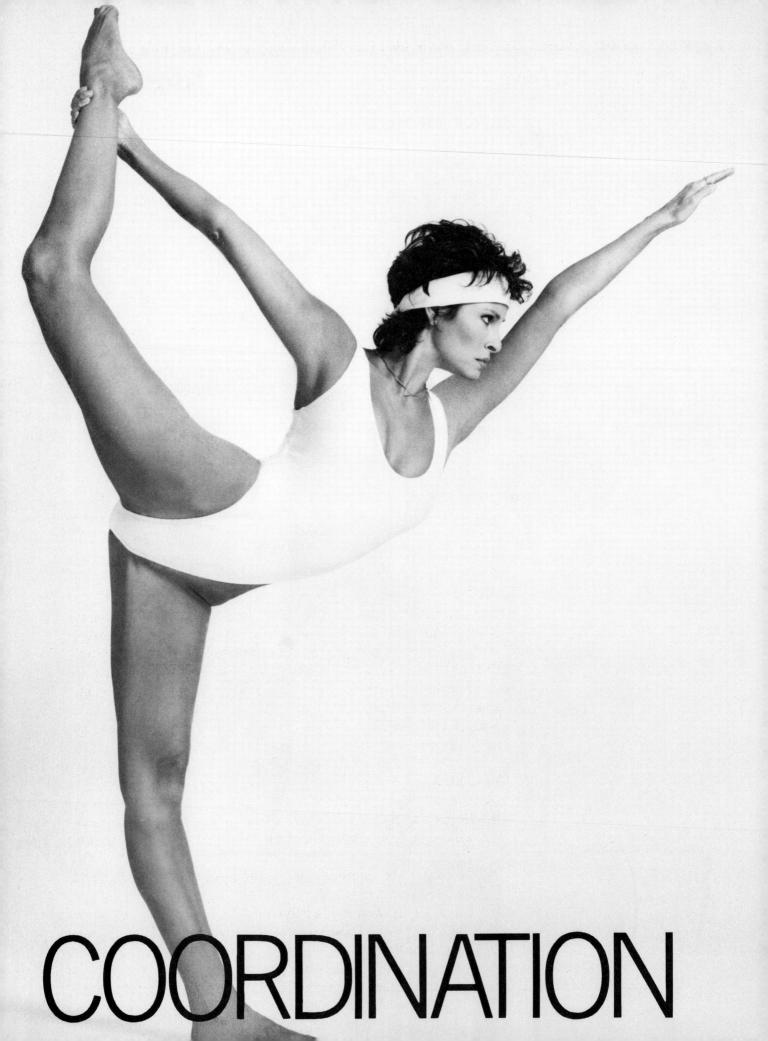

COORDINATION

Dancer's Pose

This is the most beautiful pose in the series—and possibly in yoga. Its beauty makes up for the difficulty involved in doing it. It's something worth achieving, not only for its grace but because it's a good measure of your balance, flexibility, strength, concentration . . . and all the elements we've been working on so far. In addition, it also requires *coordination,* so it ties together the other virtues you've been practicing. Once you've put the pieces of a puzzle together and made them fit, you'll create a thing of beauty and harmony.

Benefits

- Strengthens and works the muscles of the back, chest, abdomen, and legs, particularly the buttocks, upper thighs, and calves.
- Stretches and improves the flexibility of the lower spine and limbers hips and ankles.
- Expands and deepens the thorax.
- Induces concentration, coordination, balance, self-control, and determination.

Dancer's Pose

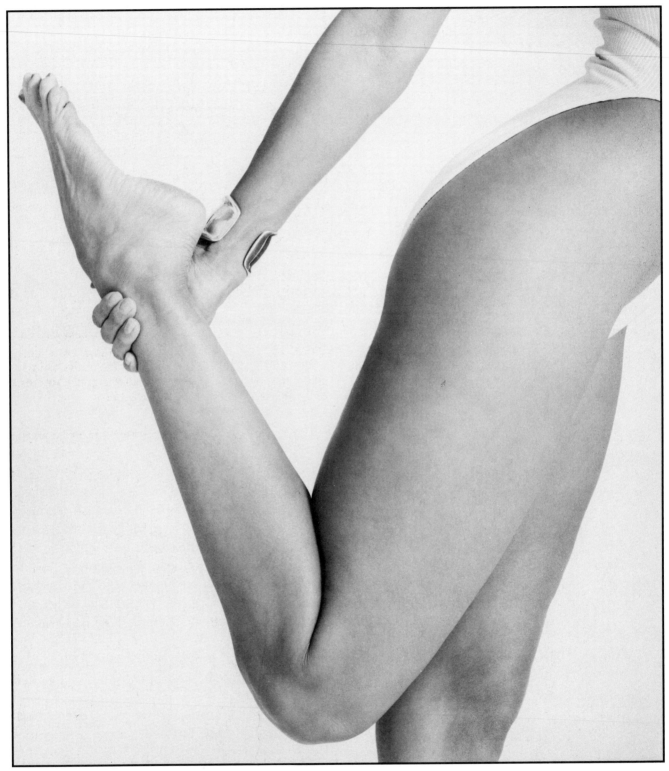

1. This shows the grip you will be using in this pose—study it a moment before beginning. Your hand should take hold of the foot slightly behind and to the side of the body. Turn your palm out and wrap the fingers and thumb around your ankle from the inside.

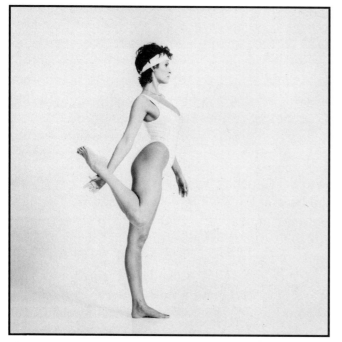

2. Now start. Find a spot ahead of you and gaze steadily at it. Shift your weight to your left foot and turn your right hand open to the side, thumb pointed backward. Bend your right leg back and prepare to grab your foot.

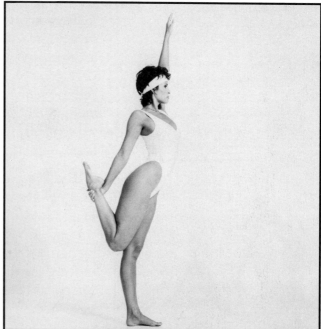

3. Place your right foot in your hand and raise your left arm straight up, fingers pointed at the ceiling. Find your balance. Settle firmly into it. Square your hips to the mirror, making sure they are even.

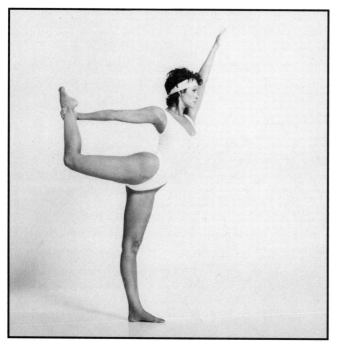

4. When you have your balance, and your standing leg is absolutely locked, inhale and begin to kick your leg backward slowly and up against your hand.

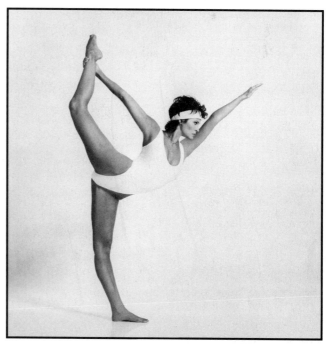

5. Continue to kick as high as you can and start to rock forward with the upper body, reaching forward with your arm. Keep your gaze fixed and hold for 10 seconds. Slowly return to the standing position and do the other side; REPEAT.

Dancer's Pose

Extra Help

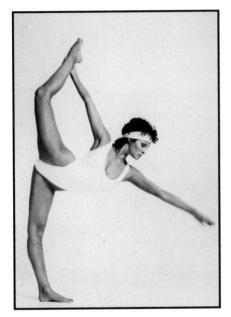

Above: *As a beginner, falling forward is not the worst thing you can do. Your weight has to be forward to get the back leg up high and increase flexibility. The abdomen should be parallel to the floor. So, if at first you fall forward, you're on the right track.*

Opposite: *For those who are more advanced, after holding the final position for 10 counts, come forward. Place your hands on the floor and try to touch your head to your leg, while kicking up as far as you can. Try for a standing split.*

1. Preparation. Don't be impatient with yourself. If you need extra time to find the correct way of holding your foot, take it. As a beginner, *getting set* is the most important thing you can do. Grip your foot, raise your arm, fix your eyes on the magic spot, square your hips, and keep your balancing leg absolutely locked and pulled tight. You simply cannot throw yourself into this pose without careful preparation, *first!* Take the extra moment to compose yourself.

2. Rocking Forward. You may feel overwhelmed at first, but this forward tilt can become rather simple with practice. The most important thing, once again, is to *keep your standing leg absolutely straight.* If you start to lose your balance, raise your arm and head higher and kick back and up more with your leg. Make sure your kicking leg does not turn out to the side. The knee should point straight back. Always kick back with a fluid motion. Don't jerk or kick suddenly. Use your buttock muscles to kick higher. And when you rock forward, reach hard with your arm toward the mirror.

3. Final Position. For those who are limber, your leg will go quite high, and you may have to adjust your hand on the leg. As you get closer to a standing split your hand will want to slide slightly farther down the leg. Let it, but keep a firm grip. However high your leg goes, your abdomen should not go lower than parallel to the floor, your weight resting slightly forward on the standing foot. Always reach forward with all your might. It's better even to fall forward occasionally when you're learning. It means you have the right approach.

Words of Encouragement

At first you may encounter difficulties, but struggle through. If you do, there's little doubt that you'll achieve this pose. Be assured your effort will be rewarded.

Did I hear you mumble something? Yes. You have a long way to go. But when you look at this photo of me, just remember that in ten years of classical ballet, I never got my leg in that position. I was thirty-five years old when I first accomplished it, after only six weeks of yoga.

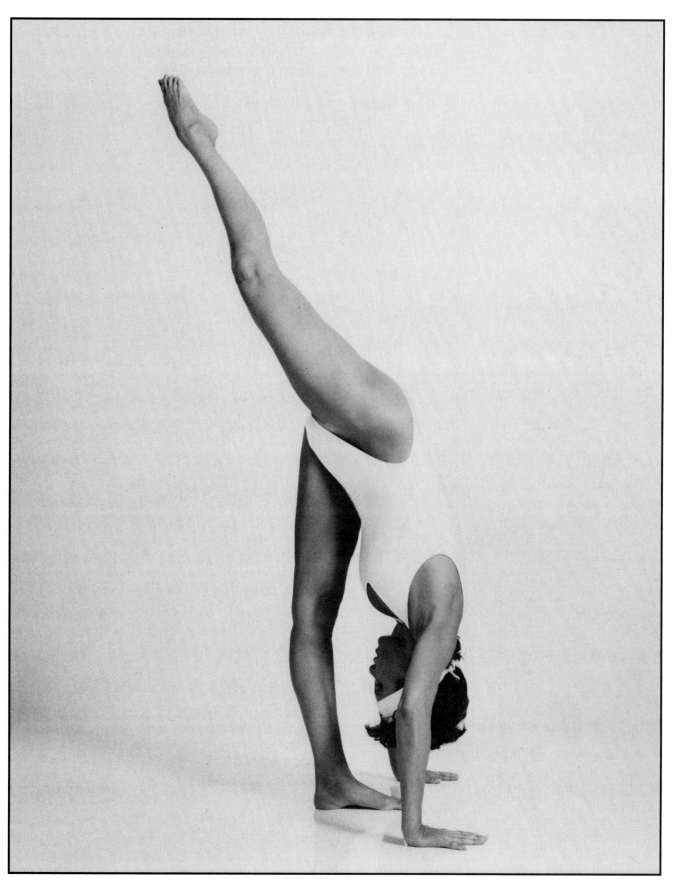

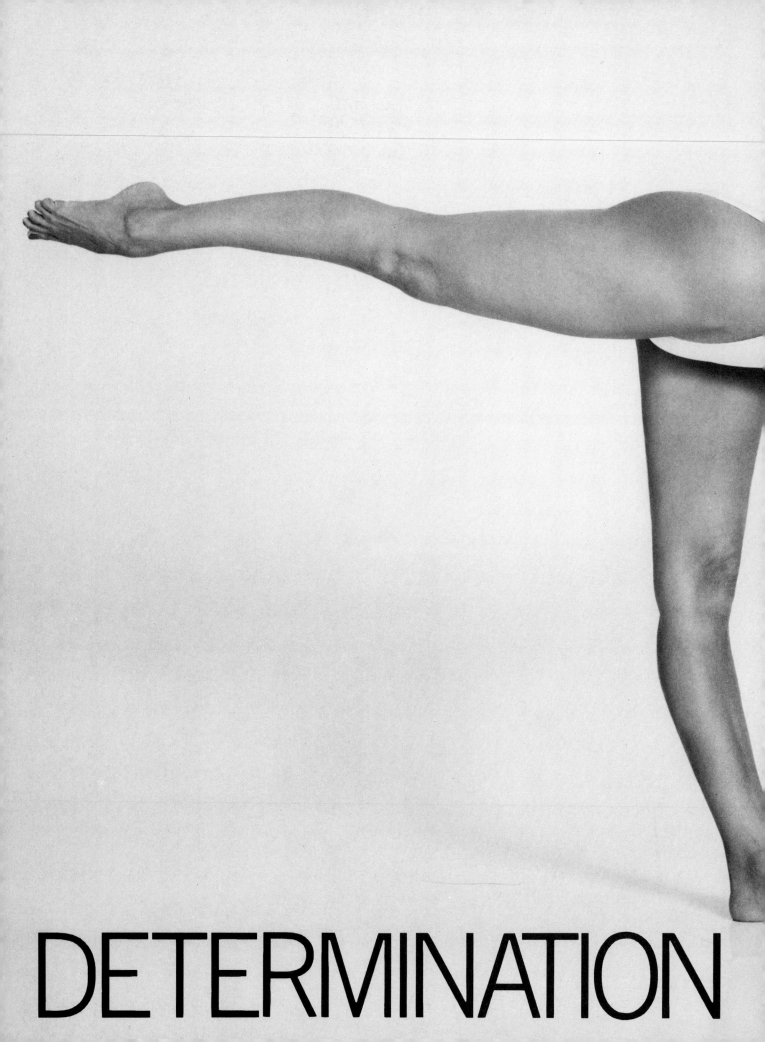

DETERMINATION

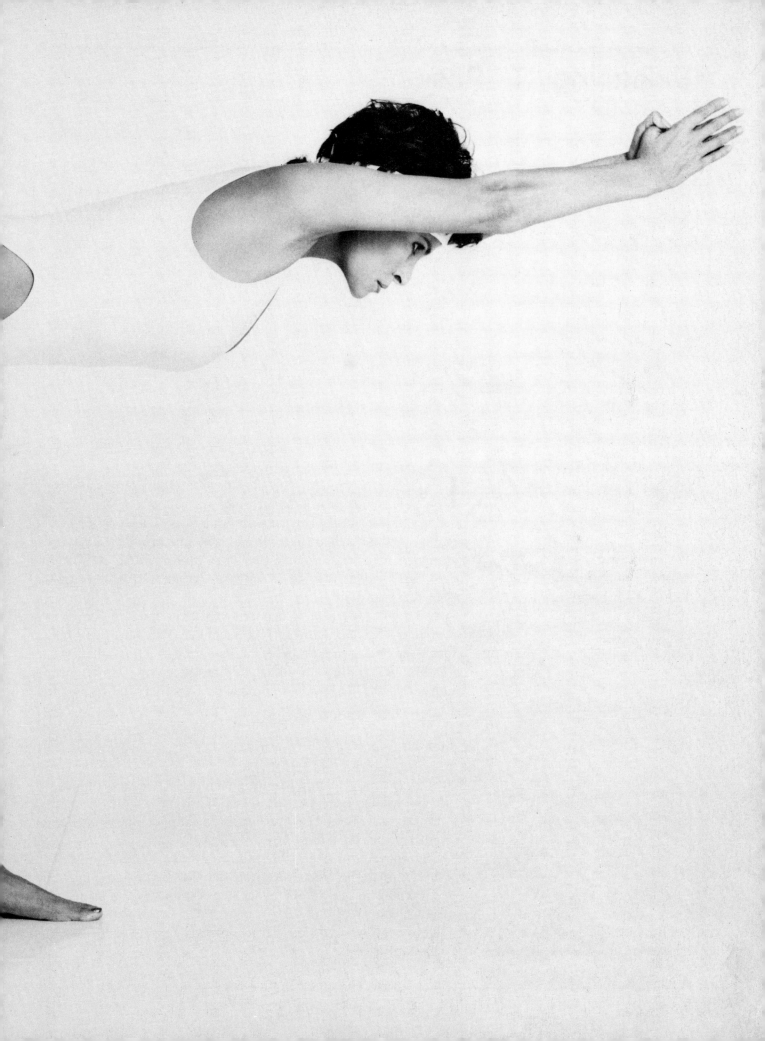

Balancing "T" Pose

We're aiming for something different. Let's call it resolve.

The key to this pose is *determination,* relaxed determination. Does that sound like a contradiction in terms? The very word "determination," after all, conjures up images of furrowed brows, pursed lips, and strident expressions. But we're aiming for something different. Let's call it resolve. Resolve to gather all your forces together and just do it . . .

"Ah," you may say, "I thought yoga was passive!" Well, it's not violent—but it's not exactly a pushover. You sweat and moan a lot in the beginning. Sometimes it's a case of doing whatever is necessary. Sort of like the adage: "When the going gets tough, the tough get going." That's the approach for beginners in this posture. Determination is *willpower.*

Benefits

- Strengthens, shapes, and adds flexibility to the legs, hips, chest, back, shoulders, upper arms, and neck.
- Works and firms the muscles of the upper back, abdomen, buttocks, and thighs.
- Stretches and limbers shoulder, hip, knee, and ankle joints.
- Builds stamina and energy, gives the heart and lungs the equivalent of an aerobic workout. Stimulates the entire cardiovascular system.
- Develops balance, concentration, and stamina and improves the posture.

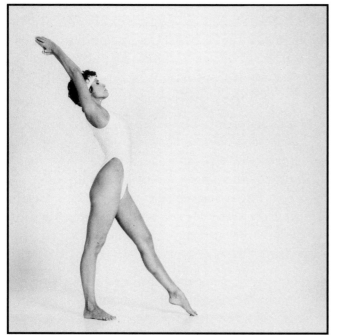

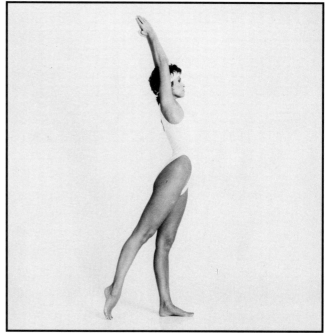

1. ■ Stand with your arms over your head, hands together as before. Reach up as high as possible. Take a deep breath, expanding the chest, and point the left foot ahead of you. Prepare to step on it.

2. ■ Step forward on an inhale and shift your weight onto the front foot.

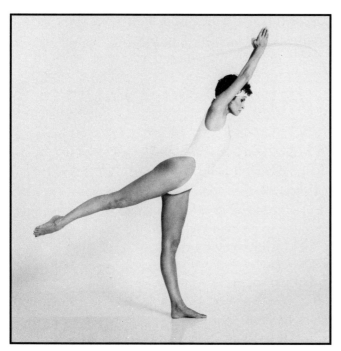

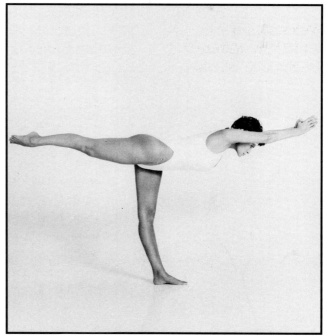

3. ■ Now, exhale and tilt your entire body forward in one piece. Make sure your standing leg is locked and that your raised leg is as stiff as a poker. Reach forward with your arms and fingertips for all you're worth.

4. ■ Come into the final position with your whole body parallel to the floor, in the shape of a "T." Hold for 10 full counts, breathing normally. If you fall out, try again. Make good use of the time. Then do the other leg, rest, and REPEAT.

Balancing "T" Pose

Extra Help

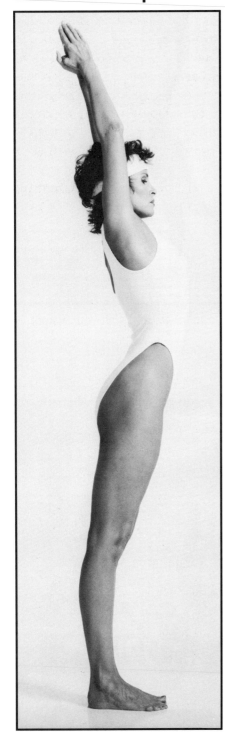

Above: *Preparation is everything. Set yourself physically and mentally before you begin. Ready, set, take a deep breath, and go.*

1. **Beginning Stance.** Follow step by step precisely the instructions given with the first two photos, with the understanding that, in particular, *how you start is how you'll finish.* As in the preceding pose, your *preparation is everything!* Also take an especially deep breath. You're going to need it.

2. **The Seesaw.** When you step forward, do so smoothly. Feel your weight *shift* onto your standing leg and try to keep your hip from twisting out. As you rock forward, control your body. Try not to analyze everything at once. Just think about *tilting* forward in a straight line from toes to fingertips. Give yourself a firm base to rock on, by keeping your standing leg absolutely locked from top to bottom. Think of rocking forward like a seesaw, your body stiff as a board, lining itself up with the floor.

3. **Holding.** When you are in position, parallel to the floor, try not to go slack. Help yourself stay stiff as a board by stretching forward with your arms as strongly as you can. Picture yourself piercing the mirror with your pointed hands and stretch your torso in the same direction. Simultaneously stretch your back leg to the wall behind you and "pierce" it also, with your pointed foot. Don't let yourself drop. Experience the pose—don't wait to get out of it.

4. **Breathing.** This is a pose with a lot of aerobic value, so your breathing will become heavy. This is good. Pant and puff unashamedly—that will smooth out in time. But above all, *do not hold your breath.*

5. **Try Again.** If you fall, just keep trying. Even if you can only manage very little. Do whatever you can do with all your might, and do it right. Good luck . . . I'll be thinking of you.

6. **In Between.** Between the left side and the right side of doing the pose, keep your arms up. I know it's hard, but do it. It may sound like one of those movies about boot camp, when the drill sergeant orders his men to stand at attention, arms extended, until they drop. But your body is nice and warmed up now, and it's time to push it a bit. It will build your stamina.

Words of Encouragement

I didn't want the ravages of old age to take over my body.

Difficult . . . very difficult, is the only way to describe this posture. No way, José, I thought when I first got a look at it. I hadn't recovered yet from the last two poses and now this! Give me a break! But I didn't want the ravages of old age—like arthritis, rheumatism, and flabby muscles—to take over my body, and I don't think you do either. So give it all you've got. Take it from me, after a few weeks of this, you'll be doing this posture with a serene resolve you never thought possible. Isn't that a delicious prospect?

Note: In addition to the other benefits listed, the Balancing "T" is also excellent for emotional stress.

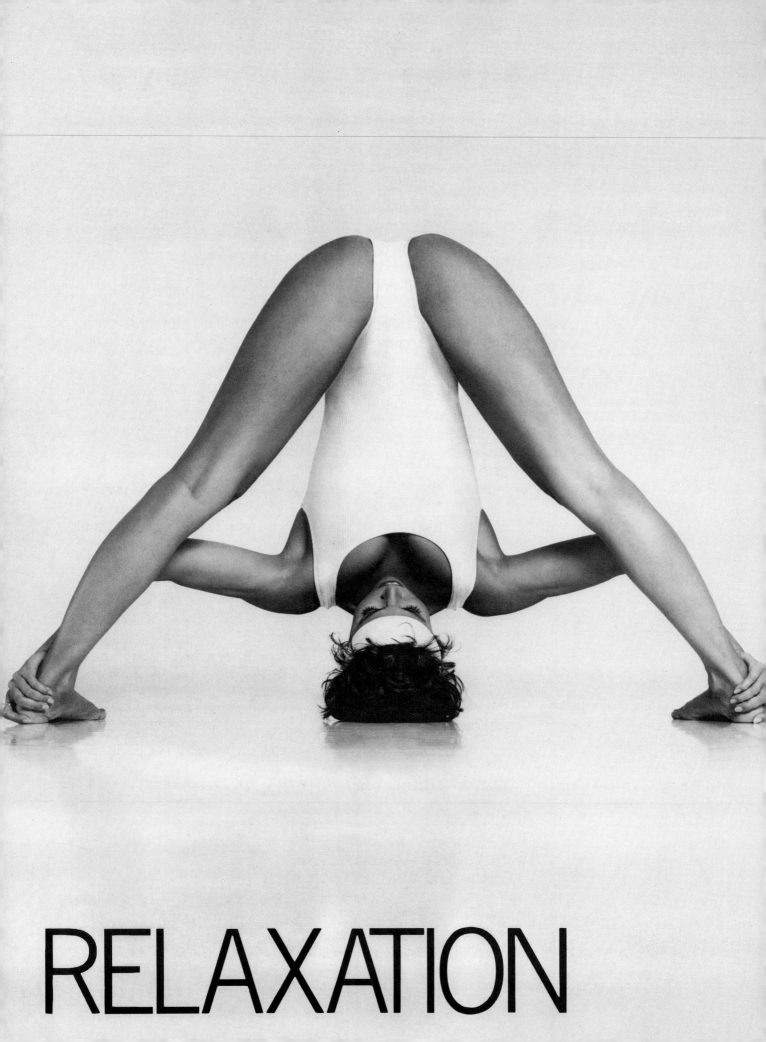

RELAXATION

Whoever heard of relaxation being an active part of exercise or body conditioning? Aren't we all supposed to work ourselves into a real frenzy to get that cardiovascular system pumping? And yet, when we're relaxed don't we always do our best? You know the answer—but still the most difficult thing for most people to do is relax. The tendency is to unconsciously hold our breath while exerting ourselves. This habit doesn't go away overnight—I myself used to be a devoted fan of turning blue from not breathing when confronted with the simplest task, much less something more demanding. On some occasions, I became absolutely catatonic and paralyzed with tension until someone kindly reminded me to breathe!

Breathing is an important part of the relaxation process. To hold the breath is to tighten the muscles and to resist impressions and sensations.

Breathing is an important part of the relaxation process. To hold the breath is to tighten the muscles and to resist impressions and sensations. Only by breathing normally and particularly *concentrating on exhalation* will you allow yourself to let go and be a part of what is happening in and around you.

Benefits

- Improves and develops flexibility.
- Tones the thigh and calf muscles.
- Stretches and strengthens the inner thighs and the ligaments, nerves, and tendons of the legs.
- Aids digestion and helps stimulate the internal organs, especially the kidneys, stomach, spleen, and intestines.

Standing "A" Stretch

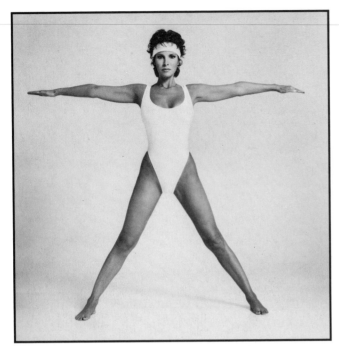

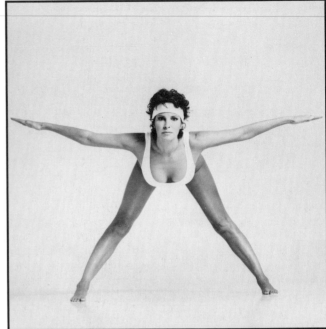

1. From a standing start with feet together, step to the right and open your arms to the side at shoulder level. Tighten your buttocks and stomach. Place your feet as far apart as possible.

2. Bend forward from the hips with the back straight, head up. Your feet should grip the floor at a slightly inward angle. Stick your bottom out in back and relax your buttocks.

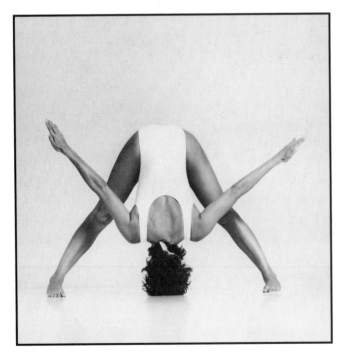

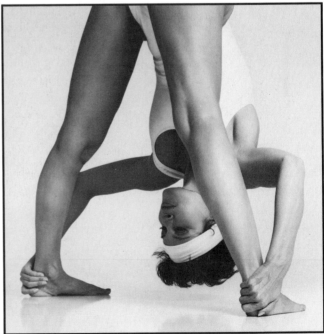

3. Exhale and go down slowly as far as you can. Try to keep your arms in this bird position, letting your body weight and gravity do the work. If possible, touch your forehead to the floor in front of you. Let yourself go!

4. When you're in your best position, slip your hands around your heels and pull yourself gently farther down. Try to get your body closer to the legs. Concentrate on exhaling—it's easier.

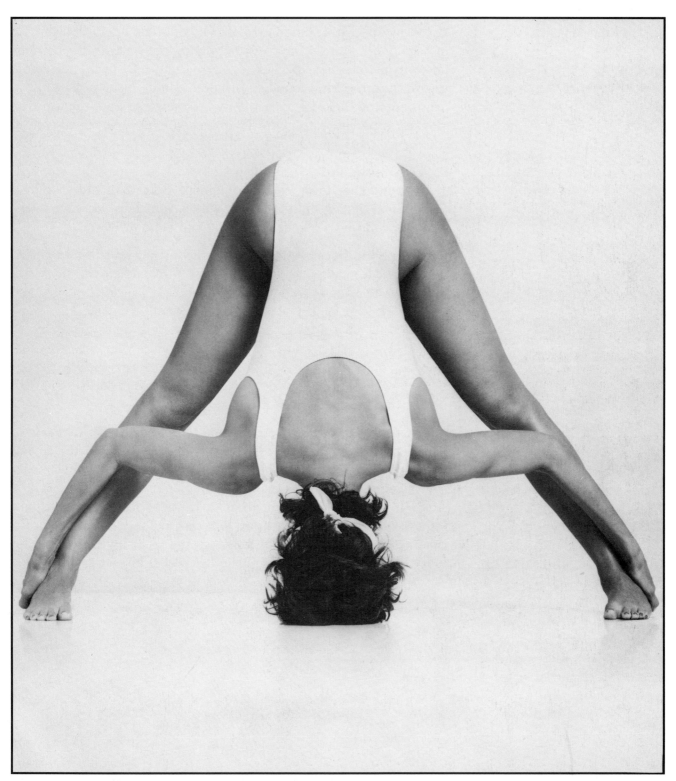

5. When your head is touching the floor, or as close as you can get, stay there for 10 seconds. *Relax* into it. As you become more limber, tip your chin inward and pull gently with your arms, so that the *top* of your head is resting on the floor. Come up *slowly* (see Extra Help), rest, and REPEAT.

Standing "A" Stretch
Extra Help

Your breakthrough will come with relaxation.

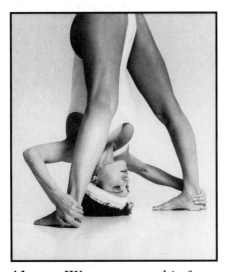

Above: *When you get this far down, eventually you may be able to pull your head through the legs, but that takes time. You may wish to close the distance between your legs, to get a better stretch.*

1. **Slipping.** First things first. If you get stuck doing this pose on a bare floor, your feet may start to slip. Try wetting the bottoms of your feet slightly, so your legs won't slide out from under you. Resin, like the kind found in a ballet studio, also works. But, of course, doing this on a carpet is best. No matter what the working surface, remember to angle your toes slightly inward to control the slip.

2. **Helping Hands.** If you feel like your tendons can't stand it, drop your hands to the floor for support. Bend your elbows to feel the pull on the back of the legs and keep your head up. Remember to stick your derriere out and up as you bend forward.

3. **Touch the Head.** As a beginner, the farther your feet are apart, the better your chance to touch your forehead to the floor. My advice is to start wide, so you get the real feel of the pose, and then work your feet in when and if it becomes too easy. Also, some of you will have a tough time with your feet quite far apart, so work on *relaxation* and *exhalation,* pull with your arms against the feet, and quietly observe the points of tension releasing in your legs, hips, and even your neck. Your breakthrough will come with relaxation. Mine did.

4. **Coming Up.** Come out of this semi-inverted posture very slowly. First, place your hands on the floor for support, then inch your feet in from the sides a few inches and roll your back up vertebra by vertebra, head last. Second, try to bring your right leg back to the left with a swift scissor motion. It's good for the inner thighs and discipline. Stand at attention, arms at the side, and rest. Remember to try to bring your legs together in a single motion after each of the poses that require the feet to be far apart.

Words of Encouragement

This is one of the most exhilarating postures in the series. It is a semi-inverted pose and therefore gives the new beginner many of the benefits of the famous Head Stand, which is much more complicated to accomplish. It is relaxing and stimulating. I always feel revitalized coming out of it and it's just what I need before attacking the next posture.

By the way, the Head Stand is not part of this series because I feel it's far too advanced for beginners. You will receive the same benefits by a combination of other postures here. So you're not missing a thing.

Below: *You always have the option of using your arms on the floor for support, either going down or coming up. You never bounce your tendons in this method—you allow them to release.*

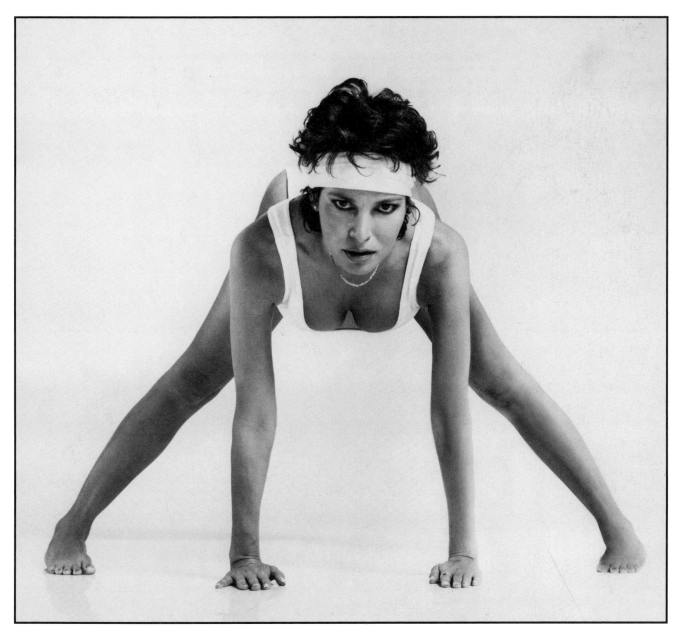

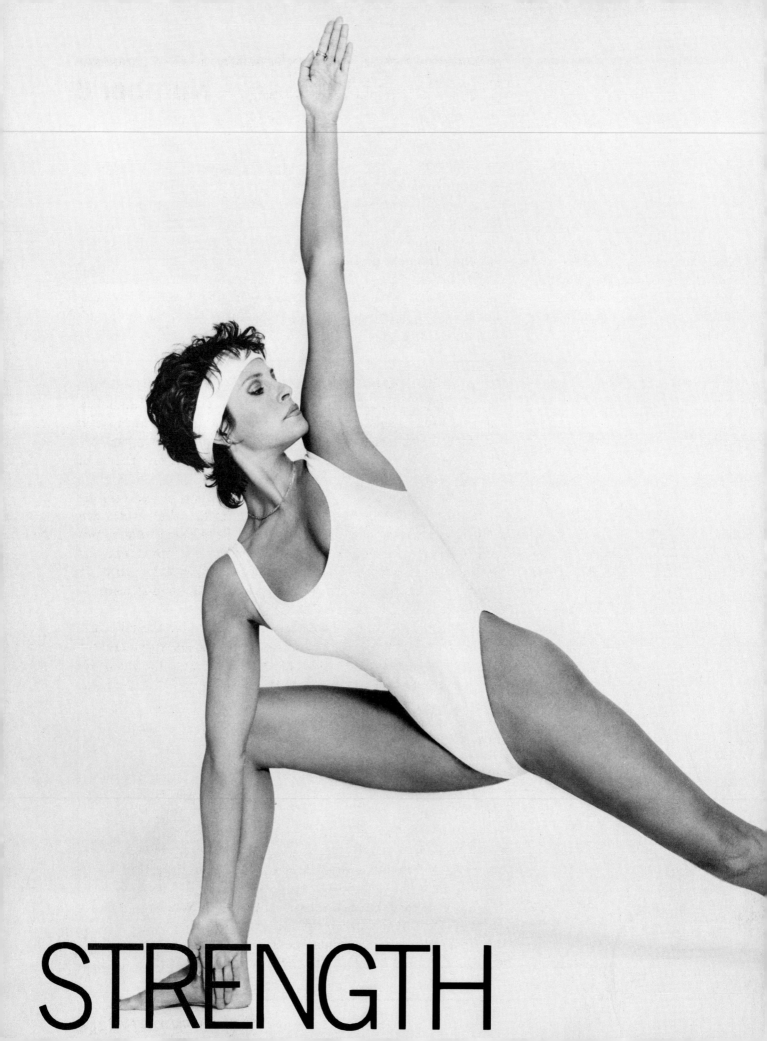

STRENGTH

The Triangle Pose   Number 9

At this point in the series, you've been progressing along from the breathing, through the stretching, concentration, balancing, coordinating, and determination—all of which combine to build your strength. By developing each of these capabilities separately and bringing them together, you can build a firm foundation of real strength.

Each of these qualities gives you the options of approaching a situation so that needless force, or the misuse of strength, can be avoided. People who tend to rely on force seem to lack two qualities: patience and confidence. They usually don't take the time to understand what's needed before deciding how to proceed. As a result, they push themselves into the fray—doing harm to themselves and others in the process.

The Triangle Pose is a position of strength—in the real sense. You support yourself by stretching and balancing, and you breathe throughout the posture to maximize your stamina. This is a beautiful posture if done correctly. Strength is a wonderful thing . . . when it supports something of beauty.

Benefits

- Works and stretches most muscles, ligaments, joints, and nerves of the body—specifically, the arms, neck, shoulders, back, hips, and legs.
- Slims the abdominals and trims the waistline.
- Helps relieve and cure backaches, stiff neck, lumbago, and rheumatism of the lower-back area by giving a lateral stretch to the spine.
- Increases and builds the strength of the ankles and corrects any minor deformity of the legs.
- Tones the spinal nervous system.
- Expands and develops the chest.

The Triangle Pose

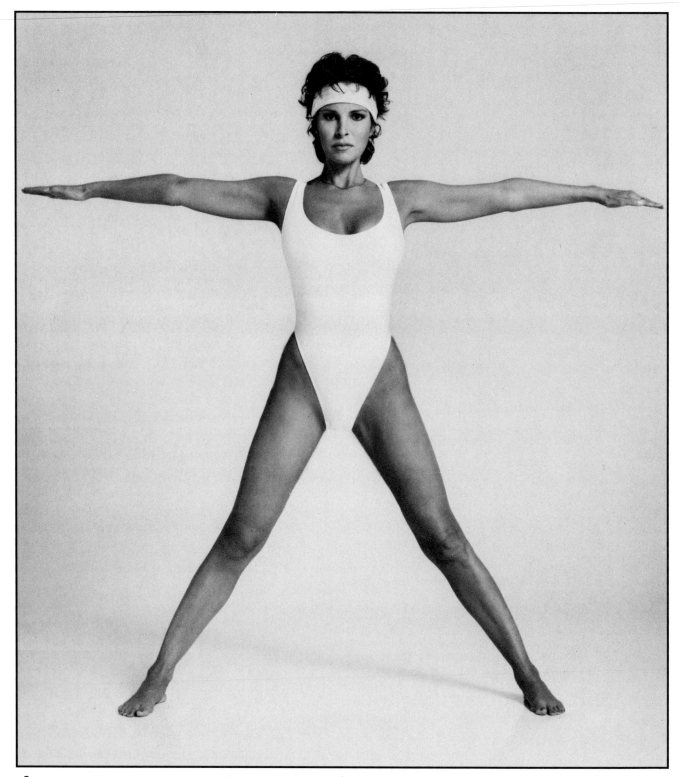

1. From a standing start with your feet together and arms over the head, step to the right in a nice wide stance, lowering the arms to shoulder level. Tuck in your hips and stomach and keep your shoulders back and down.

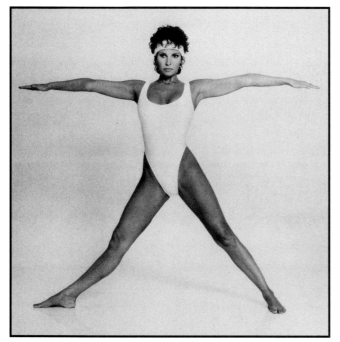

2. Simply turn your right foot to the side at a 90-degree angle to the other foot. Keep your hips facing front.

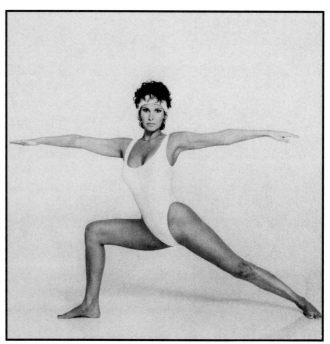

3. Now, bend your right knee over the right foot and lunge to the side slowly with control until your thigh is parallel to the floor.

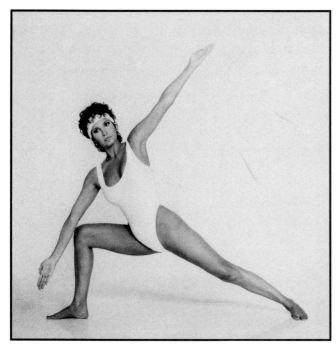

4. At this point, tilt your upper body and arms in one line toward the bent leg. Stretch your top arm up and don't let your hips rise. Stay facing the mirror and check your movement.

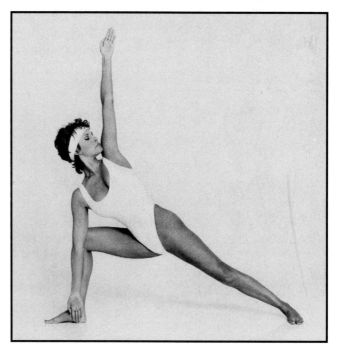

5. Continue tilting until your hand reaches this position (see Extra Help). Turn your face to your raised shoulder. Push your hips forward and draw yourself up out of your torso. Hold for 10 counts. Breathe normally. Come back up to step 1, do the other side. Rest, and REPEAT.

The Triangle Pose

Extra Help

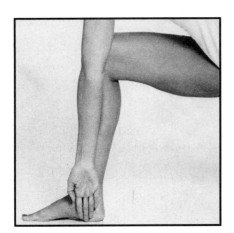

Above: *This is the correct hand position. The fingers should barely touch the floor and no weight should rest on the fingertips. Reach to the ceiling with your raised arm and press back against the knee with the other.*

1. The Lunge. When you take your first lunge onto one leg, there are several things to coordinate. Keep the bottom of your thigh parallel to the floor and feel the thigh muscle holding you. Sit into it and tighten your buttocks. This is your seat of power. *Make sure your hips don't rise up when you raise your arm. Keep them even.* And of course, the extended leg should be absolutely straight and locked.

2. Arms. While tilting your arms over, don't allow your body to collapse or sink down. Reach with your top arm like crazy and press forward with the hips. *Do not lean on your fingers by the ankle. Keep reaching up* throughout the pose.

3. Hand Position. The exact hand position by the foot depends on the person. It can be farther forward of the ankle, or even by the toes. The object is to make a straight line with the arms between the fingertips. Experiment at first and find the best point. Remember to press back against the bent knee with your elbow.

4. Head Twist. Sometimes the head just doesn't seem to want to turn around. Alright, do your best and don't worry about it. It will come with practice. Try, but don't force it.

5. Breathing. I found the key to this posture was to concentrate on my breathing and not to panic. You have a lot more reserve strength at your disposal than you imagine. Strike the pose and forget about counting the seconds until you can get out of it. Try just breathing while you're in it and *voilà!*, pretty soon you're holding for the full count and more.

Words of Encouragement

It took me a long time to build strength and stamina in this pose. I could get into it alright, but staying there was another story.

There's so much to think about on this one, while your thigh is quivering and you're running out of gas, that you may be tempted to pack it in. Press on. Do the best you can and miraculously your strength grows. But stick with it. Don't get discouraged. Even a nonviolent approach takes consistent effort.

Below: *Getting into it is one thing—staying is another. Even a nonviolent approach takes consistent effort.*

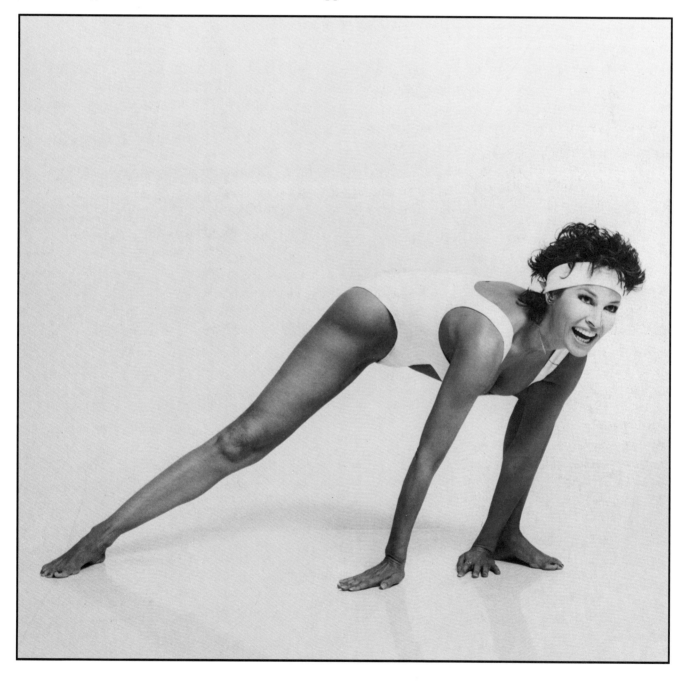

TRANSITION

Standing "A" Head to Knee

Number 10

After the exertion spent on the Triangle Pose, you deserve to equalize the energy flow again and effect a recovery. The Standing "A" is simple and straightforward, and since it is an easier posture than others, some people don't make much effort. Once again, it's back to the foolish philosophy of "No pain, no gain." Wrong!

The Standing "A" also serves as a link between the last pose and the one ahead, allowing you—like a bridge in a musical score—to make a smooth transition into a different movement. Transitions make possible the successful blending of different elements. They are sometimes perceived as trivial, but without them we'd have no way to connect things together. Everything would be a cul de sac, a dead end. Think about it—they're not a detail, they're a necessity.

Benefits

- Improves the elasticity of the spine, hip joints, and legs.
- Tones and stretches the muscles, ligaments, and nerves of the thighs and calves.
- Tightens and firms the buttocks and thighs.
- Removes superfluous fat from the waistline.
- Helps and improves functioning of the abdominal organs, as well as the kidneys.

Standing "A" Head to Knee

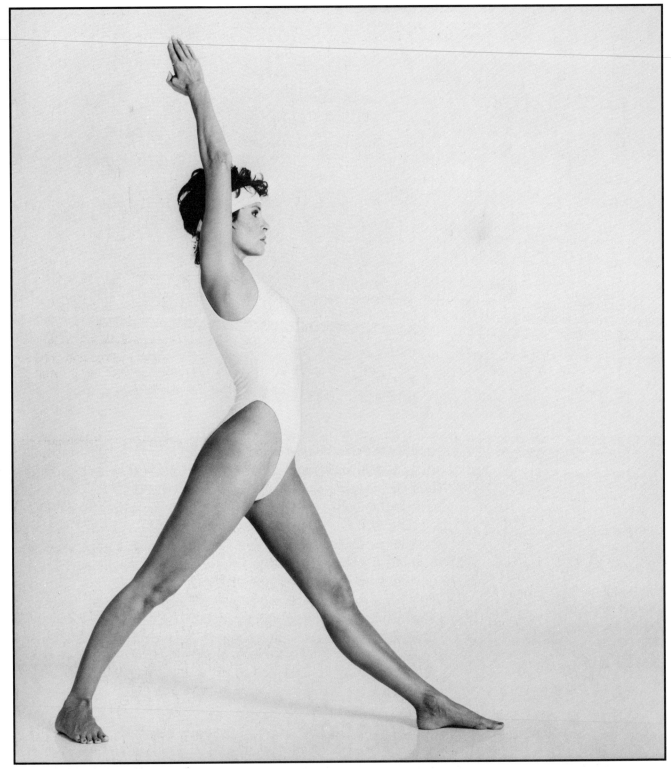

1. Start this pose the same way as the last one: from a standing position with your arms over the head, step to a wide stance keeping the arms up; turn your right foot to the side. Then, turn your head and your upper body to the same direction.

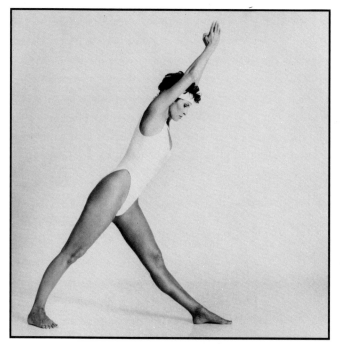

2. Exhale and start to bend forward from the hips. Keep your body in one line over the forward leg.

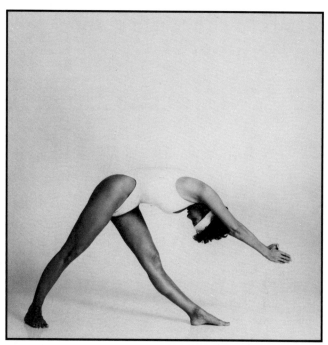

3. Tuck your chin in tightly to your chest and continue forward. Aim for the knee with your head. Keep your legs straight and knees locked.

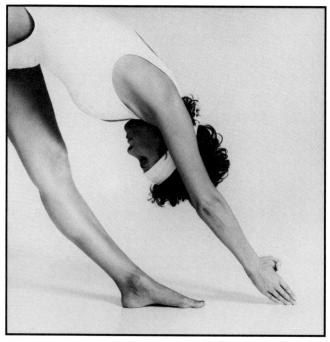

4. When your fingertips touch the floor, don't stop. Exhale and proceed farther.

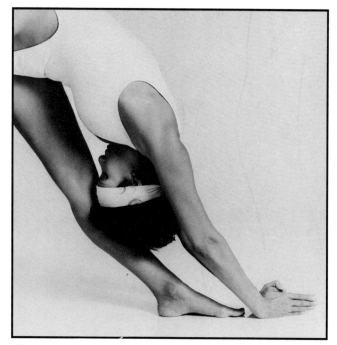

5. Curl your body inward and place your forehead on the knee. Rest the sides of your hands on the floor if you can, or hold on to your leg. Stay in the pose for 10 seconds, breathing normally. Return to step 1, do the other side, rest, and REPEAT.

Standing "A" Head to Knee

Extra Help

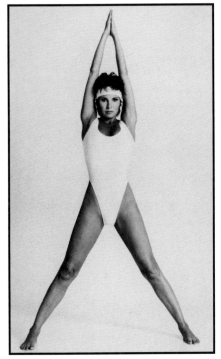

Above: *This is the starting position, with the legs apart. Buttocks should be tight, stomach in, and reach for the ceiling. Starting right is important—your body knows the difference.*

1. Head to Knee. The first priority, above everything else in this posture, is to *touch the head to the knee.* Just concentrate on that before making any other adjustments. *Curl your chin to your chest, round your back, and aim for the knee.* It's this curving action that helps the kidneys. Dear beginner, if you really need to bend your knee to make the connection, do so for the first few days. Then slowly begin pressing back against the knee to straighten it when your back gains flexibility. This may take some time. So don't give up easily.

2. Stay and Breathe. The benefits in this pose come from placing the head on the knee and staying there. Believe it or not, your back and legs will release if you do nothing else but that and concentrate on exhalation!

3. Straighten Legs. After a few days, when you feel the limberness coming, press back on your knee with your hand to help straighten your leg. You should feel a pull on the back of your leg—that's alright. Continue to exhale and stretch. Don't force it, however, there's no need. You will progress gradually and steadily with patience and persistence.

4. Even Hips. When your head is finally on your straight knee, then you can concern yourself with evening your hips. Check in a mirror to see if one is higher than the other. Then swivel them around.

5. Last Details. Before going forward, check to see that your feet are in one line, and your legs are absolutely straight. If you cannot bend forward very far, just do the best you can. If your hands don't touch the floor in front of you, rest them on your legs. But give your best effort and keep your chin tucked in and your head toward that knee.

Words of Encouragement

This pose used to puzzle me until I found out what good therapy it is for the kidneys. Then I was a lot more careful about doing it precisely. It's also a great refresher and signals the gearing down of the standing postures. Go with it.

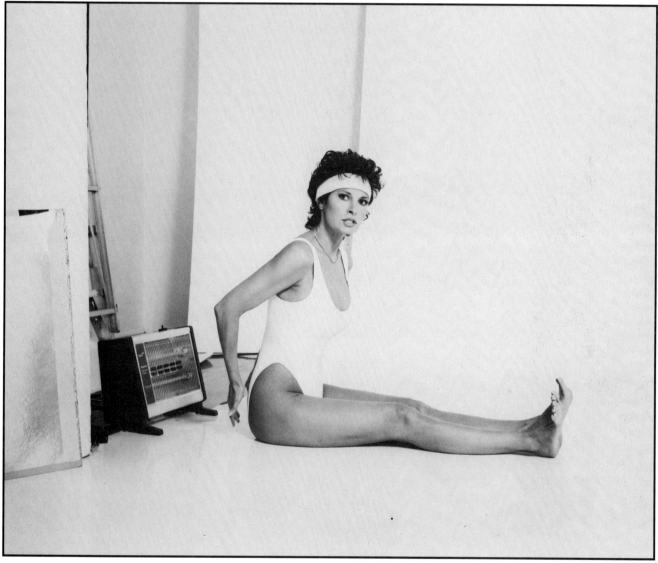

Above: *Heating up your backside can be great when working in a chilly room.*

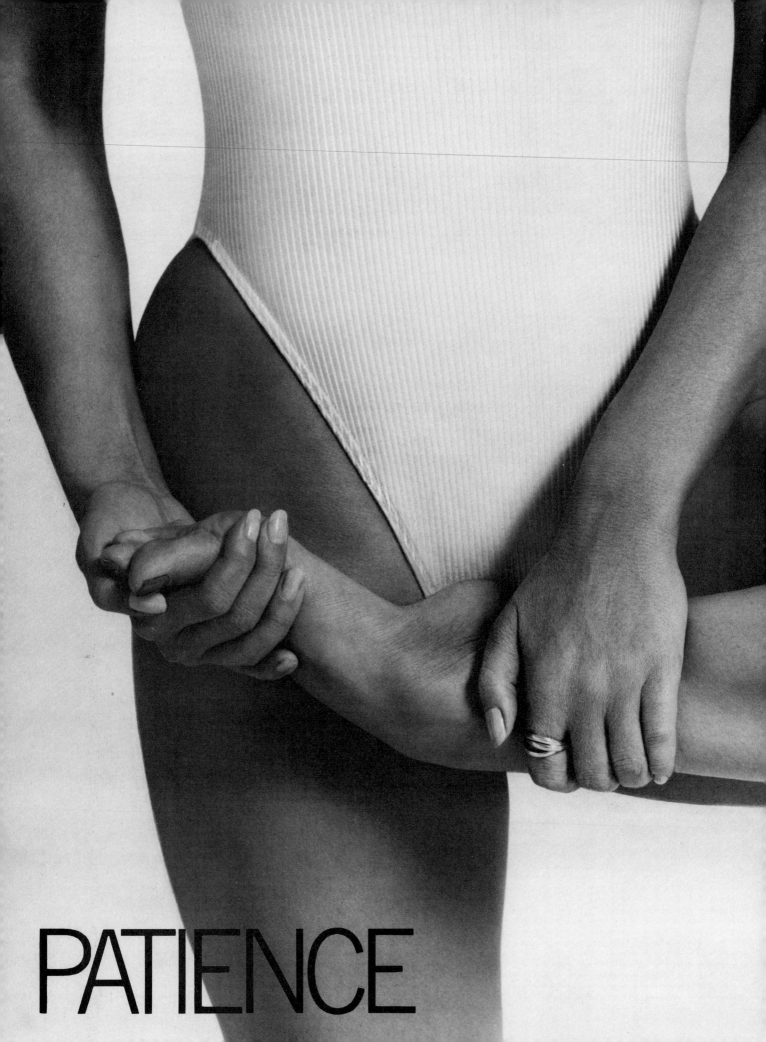

PATIENCE

Tree Pose   Number 11

W hat we are trying to develop in this posture is confidence and persistence in the face of problems and obstacles. If you practice it patiently, things do seem to fall into place. Patience can be an elusive quality often confused with waiting—and although waiting requires patience, it's not quite the same thing. I think patience describes your *mental attitude* while you wait.

To develop patience you must calmly resist all ploys that conspire to discourage you—only this time, the enemy is not an outside force . . . it's within. You've got to fight off every inner demon that your psyche can throw in the way, from vanity to lack of faith and confidence. Beware of anger, fear, even stupidity. Funnily enough, when you meet these demons, you'll probably fail to recognize them—after all, they look and sound so much like you!

"Genius is nothing but a greater aptitude for patience," said the French philosopher Georges de Buffon. And St. Francis of Assisi said, "Where there is patience and humility, there is neither anger or vexation." So hang in there—with such lofty encouragement, you can't go wrong!

Benefits

- Strengthens, tones, and increases the flexibility of the legs— specifically limbers the ankle, knee, and hip joints.
- Helps prevent varicose veins by improving blood circulation in the legs.
- Improves concentration and sense of balance and helps correct and achieve a better posture.

Tree Pose

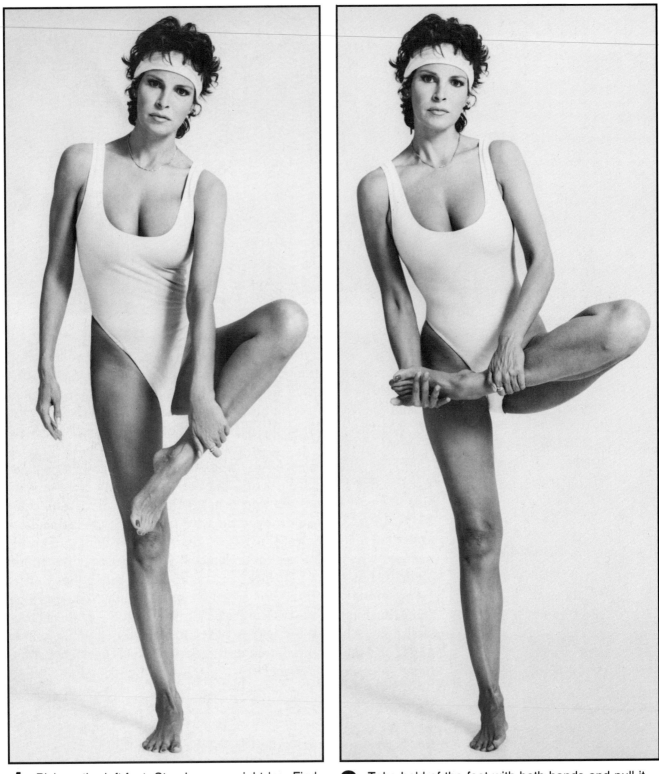

1. Pick up the left foot. Stand on your right leg. Find a spot and fix your eyes on it for the duration of the posture.

2. Take hold of the foot with both hands and pull it high up the opposite leg. Place the left foot into the upturned palm of your right hand.

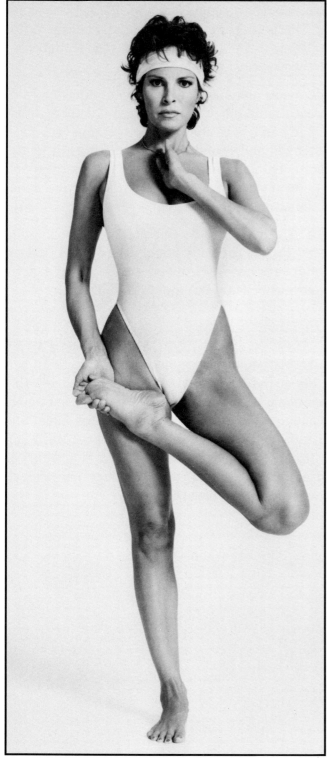

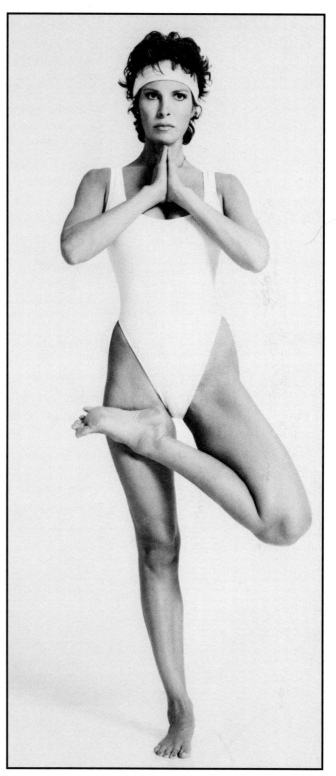

3. Hold your leg in this high position and press the knee down. The foot should rest against the upper thigh. Fix your eyes to your spot and raise your left hand to your chest, in the half-prayer position.

4. Lift your torso, tuck in your hips and place your other hand in the prayer position. Keep your back straight and your shoulders down. Relax and hold for 10 counts, breathing normally. Drop the leg down, and do the other side. Rest, and REPEAT.

Tree Pose

Extra Help

Half a prayer is better than no prayer at all!

Opposite: *Sometimes you just have a goofy day, and you can't steady yourself—laugh and keep going. It happens to the best of us.*

1. Foot Up. It's truly hard for some people to lift their foot high up the standing leg. This is fairly common—especially among men—and comes from stiffness in the knees and hips. You'll limber up with practice. Don't worry. Just keep at it.

2. Half Prayer. If you're anxious that once you manage to pull your foot up with both hands, it won't stay there, don't be. Just keep holding with one hand as in step 3, keep pressing your knee down, tighten your hips, and remain in the half prayer for the count. Half a prayer is better than no prayer at all! Test yourself from time to time to see if you can hold it there without your hand. It may take some time, so try to be patient with yourself.

3. Side Check. It's very helpful to do this pose with your profile to the mirror, so that you can correct yourself. Here's what to look for: both knees should be in one line, and your back straight; don't sway back, tuck your buttocks under, and hold yourself erect.

Words of Encouragement

At first it seems that you are being asked to become a human pretzel. How can this be natural, you may well ask. And yet, this is similar to the position that the fetus rests in while in the womb, awaiting birth. It is only after years of disuse that the knees and hips become rigid and eventually cause us to be practically immobile in old age from arthritis, rheumatism, etc. So strange as it may seem, "pretzel legs" are very natural, healthy, and, in fact, wonderful insurance against the ravages of time.

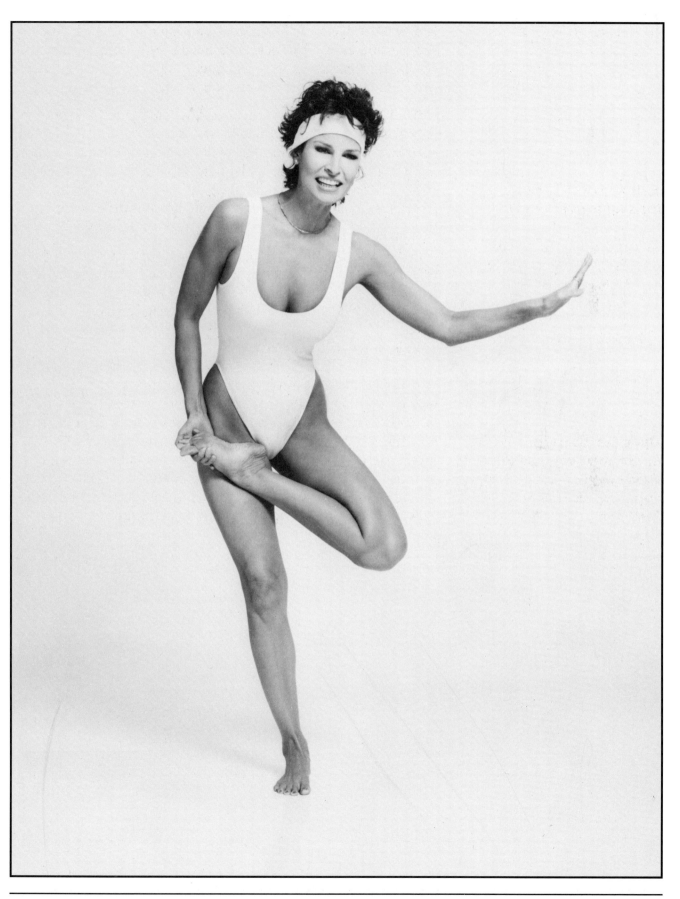

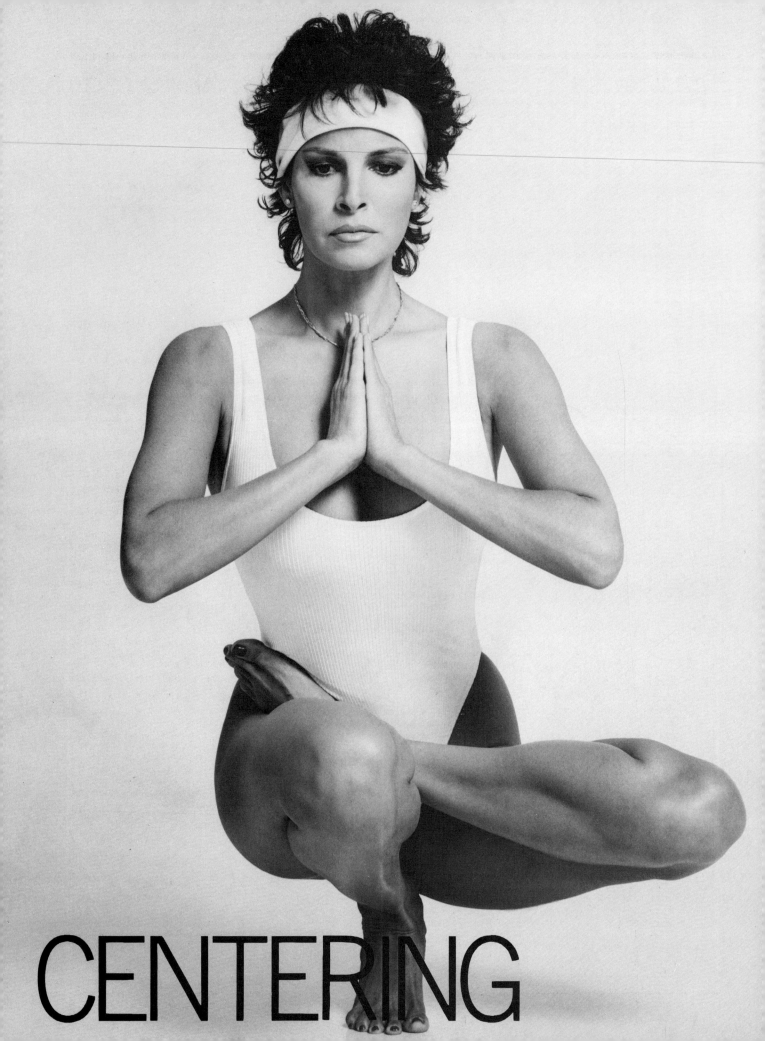

CENTERING

Everyone longs to have "a little peace and quiet"; yet every day millions of Americans suffer from tension headaches and related back pains—the pressures are too great. Well, here's your chance to have your own portable oasis to carry around with you, wherever you go—in a word, your own center.

When you discover your own center, everything else follows. The pains and headaches slip away . . . the cellulite disappears from your flesh . . . your muscles define themselves on your body . . . and you feel and look great. Your instincts will be clearer, your judgments more accurate. Your newly found confidence will act like an alchemist, turning anxiety into peace of mind—like turning lead into gold.

The object of the Toe Stand is to help you find and hold your center. The center is located where your energy runs through your spine, up the back of your neck, into your brain. It will seem to give you buoyancy and lightness, as though the atmosphere around you were water. You are floating there, in a sea of air, in your fixed pose. Other concerns fade away and you are absolutely still, except for your breathing, which comes and goes on its own.

Up until now, you've been getting through any way you can, by hook or crook. Good! Now, with this pose, it's time for the fidgeting to stop.

In the Toe Stand you are required to be absolutely still and completely eliminate any superficial movement, including blinking; choose a spot and fix your gaze. If you lose your balance it doesn't matter—just *do not lose your spot*. Your body will correct itself. Do not budge. Obey the instructions step by step. Simply do not question anything. The less you think, the better you'll *do*.

Benefits

- Works especially on the hip, knee, and ankle joints.
- Tones the spine and abdomen.
- Improves coordination, balance, and patience.
- Helps cure or prevent rheumatism of the legs.

Toe Stand

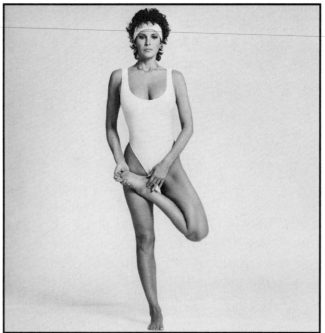

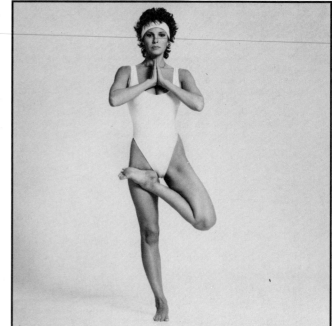

1. Stand on your right leg and bring your other foot up high on the opposite leg as in the previous pose. Fix your eyes on one point in front of you and find your balance.

2. Bring your hands together in the prayer position. Since you're already warmed up to do this, you should be able to assume this final position more easily—knee down, standing leg locked, hips tucked, etc.

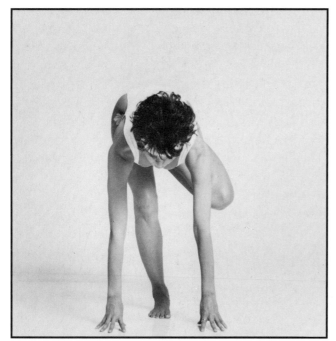

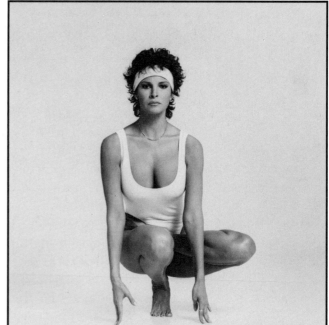

5. When you have to, reach forward and touch the floor to support yourself the rest of the way down. Do not collapse, however. Use control and strength as much as possible.

6. Once your hips are resting *lightly* on your heels, straighten your back again and find an eye spot on the floor, a few feet in front of you. This helps you maintain balance. Try to center your spine.

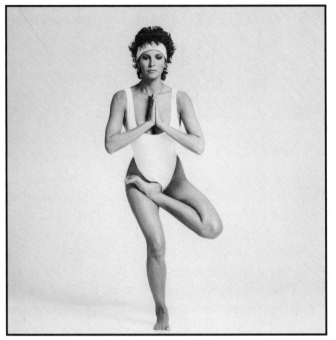

3. This time, very slowly, bend your straight leg and start to lower yourself down.

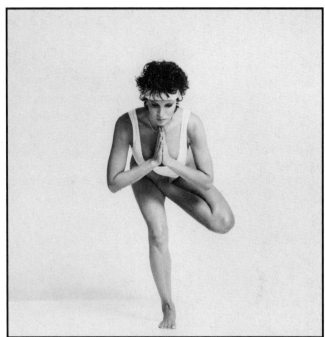

4. Bend forward as you go, but remain straight for as long as possible and keep your hands together. Work your leg muscles.

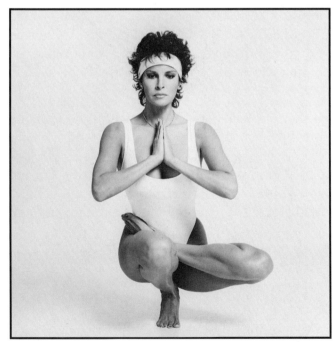

7. Now ease your fingertips off the floor. First, one hand, then the other. Bring hands together again in prayer position. Hold for 10 counts, never letting your eyes stray from their spot.

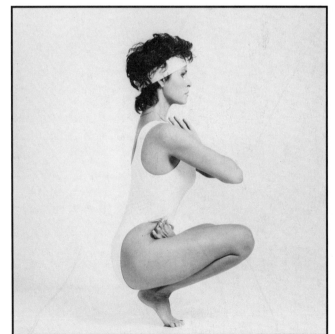

8. From profile, your back should be straight. Imagine that your breath is lifting your spine with each inhalation and suspending you from the top of your head. Come up the same way you went down, do the other leg, rest and *do not repeat.*

Toe Stand

Extra Help

1. Getting Down. Just when you thought you'd had enough trouble keeping your leg on your thigh, you're confronted with how you can possibly get down on one leg from such a high perch! The answer is simply by bending your knee! It's so obvious that you overlooked it because you've gotten overimpressed with the difficult appearance of this pose. Frankly, it took me a while to lick this one myself. But for starters, just bend your standing knee and go down slowly. You'll be fine.

2. Gaze Balance. Once down, I use my gaze to support me in balance. By this time, you must know that concentration on one spot is *key* to balance, but I found a new twist on the fixed gaze technique for this pose. First, I lock my eyes on a point on the floor, about 3 feet ahead of me. Then I use the image of a fine string that runs from my gaze to the spot on the floor. When I find my center of balance, I make believe that the string becomes solid and is supporting me there, like a fine brace or the foot on the back of a picture frame.

3. Arm Balance. You can also use your arms to hold your balance. If you find yourself fanning the air around you in an attempt to locate your center, this is fine. It's a natural instinct and may help you on your way.

4. Up Again (Coming Up). This pose is not over until you're standing up straight again. Here's what to do: put your hands on the floor in front of you and *push,* while lifting your torso. Do exactly the same motion in reverse as when you went down. Look at step 5.

5. More Advanced. After you get used to coming down more smoothly, using your hands on the floor, make an attempt to do it "without hands" all the way down. This is the ideal. So far, I've never managed to do this myself. Almost, but not quite. I'm not giving up now though, when I'm so close. Once down, I can balance for 20 seconds. When I started out I used to fall flat on my bottom.

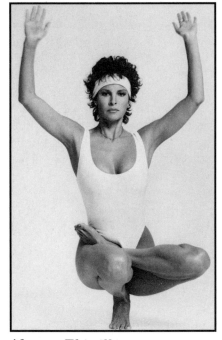

Above: *This illustrates one way to steady yourself when you are finding your balance. (See paragraph 3.)*

Words of Encouragement

The Toe Stand is a real challenge to your skeptical nature. It dares you to give it a try. But once you learn to master it, you will have found your center.

The center of your energy comes from the base of your spine. This "pipeline to paradise" may be a bit rusty at first, but you won't mind. You'll just want a return ticket. Each time you revisit, it becomes more polished, until a bright clear stream of energy travels through it freely to the top of your head. You could say it's a "nice" feeling—that's an understatement.

Below: *Yet another graceful moment spent waving my arms around like a traffic cop, trying hard not to fall on my bottom!*

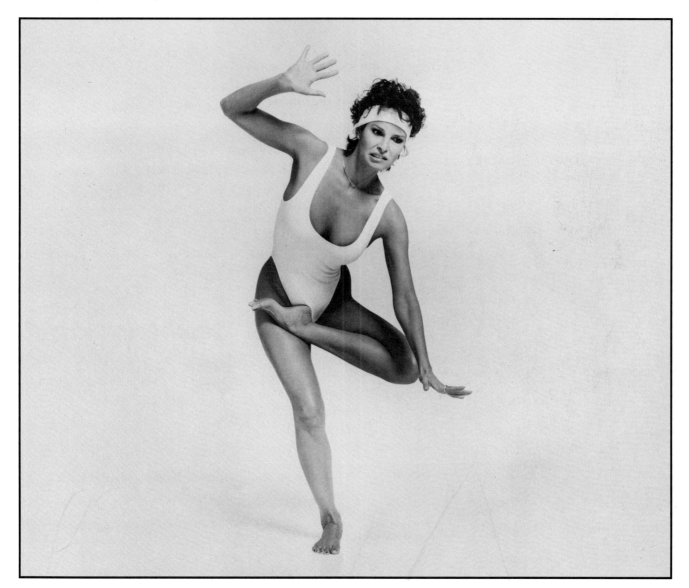

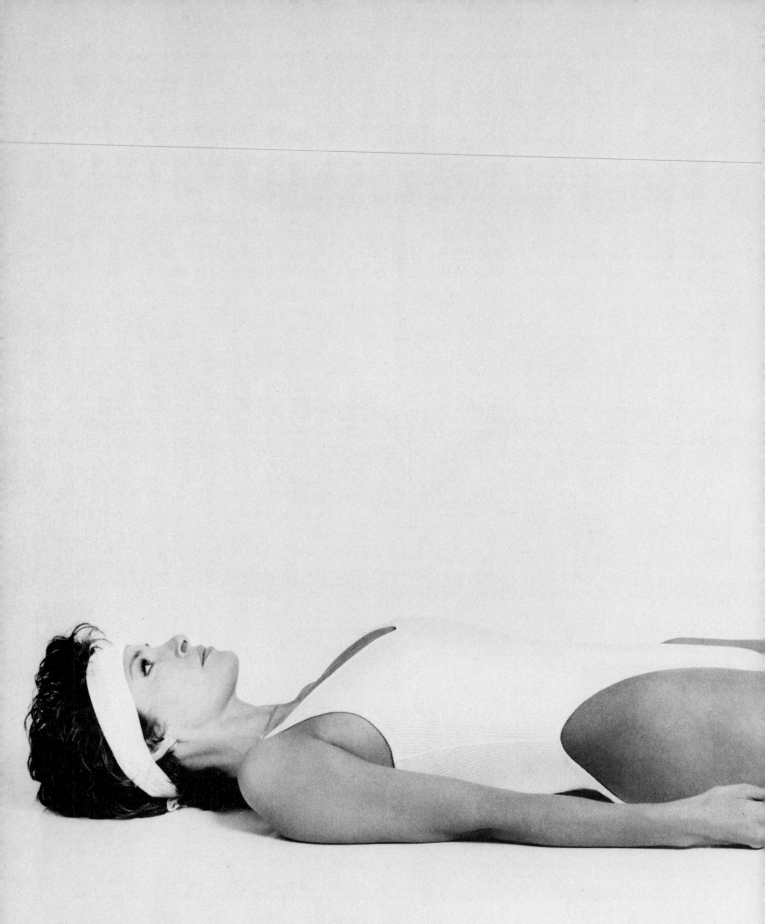

STILLNESS

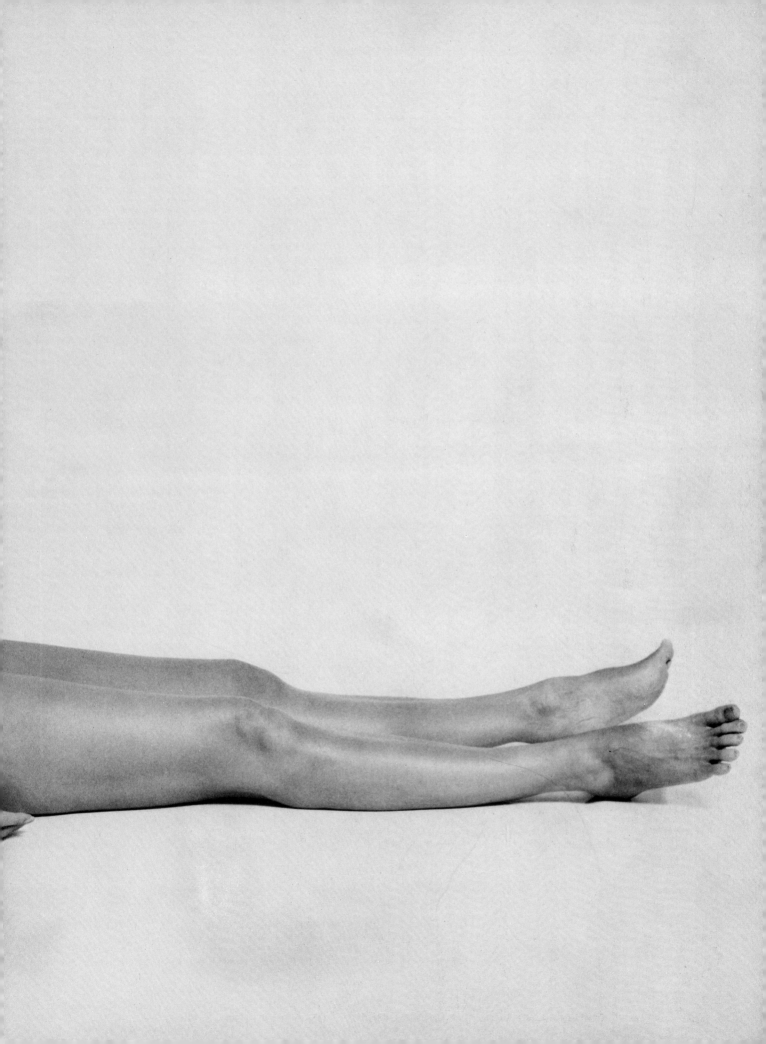

Dead Man's Pose

Stop! Don't do anything. Can you just let go? . . . Give up? . . . Surrender even for a few moments? . . . Can you stay out of your own way, both mentally and physically, and give yourself over to the moment?

Sounds easy enough. But you have an urge to participate in the process, don't you? Your mind is looking around for something to *do!*

To stop, to submit to stillness, to release all tension and relax is the hardest thing you'll ever be asked *not* to do. But that's the key to this pose and you cannot accomplish it any other way.

Everything thus far has been in preparation for, and leading up to, this. So now that you're here, you have one chance to do absolutely *nothing*.

Benefits

- Totally relaxes and rests the mind and body.
- Kills stress.
- Removes any fatigue or strain caused by the previous postures.
- Reduces respiration and pulse rate back to normal.

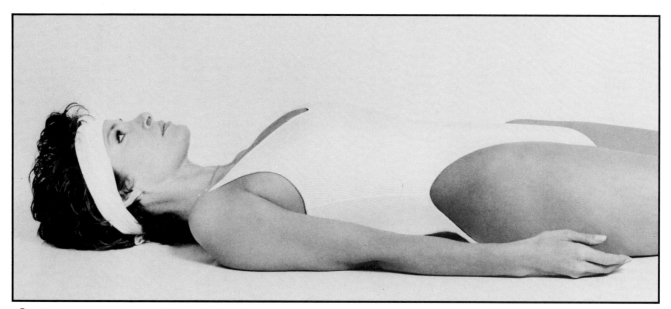

1. Relax on your back. You've earned it. Your feet loose, arms at the sides, palms slightly upwards. Just relax, let your body melt into the floor. No tension. No effort. Some people prefer to rest their hands on their abdomen and feel the flow of the breath more physically. This is your chance to do and think nothing for 3 full minutes before we continue. Don't miss it!

Note: Before you lie down, spread a mat or a towel out so you can go right into the next posture.

Extra Help

1. Eyes. While you're resting keep your eyes *open*. Don't drift off into never-never land. It's not time to sleep yet. This drowsy feeling is good because it's a sure sign of released tension. But don't give in to it so soon. I know, you haven't felt so relaxed in a long time and you'd love to just fall asleep now. But hold off. You'll see that you can revitalize yourself easier when tension is gone, so keep your eyes open—the best is yet to come.

Words of Encouragement

Many different yoga routines start with this pose as an aid to quiet the mind before starting the postures. But this method uses Deep Breathing to prepare for the standing postures and the Dead Man's Pose as the prize at the end of your effort.

I prefer it this way because I have a lot of pressure in my work and after the standing postures I am much more able to release my tensions and my relaxation is more complete. Having the Dead Man's Pose at this point in the sequence of postures serves two purposes: to relax me from tension more fully and to revive me for the second half of the routine. You see, there is a method to the madness!

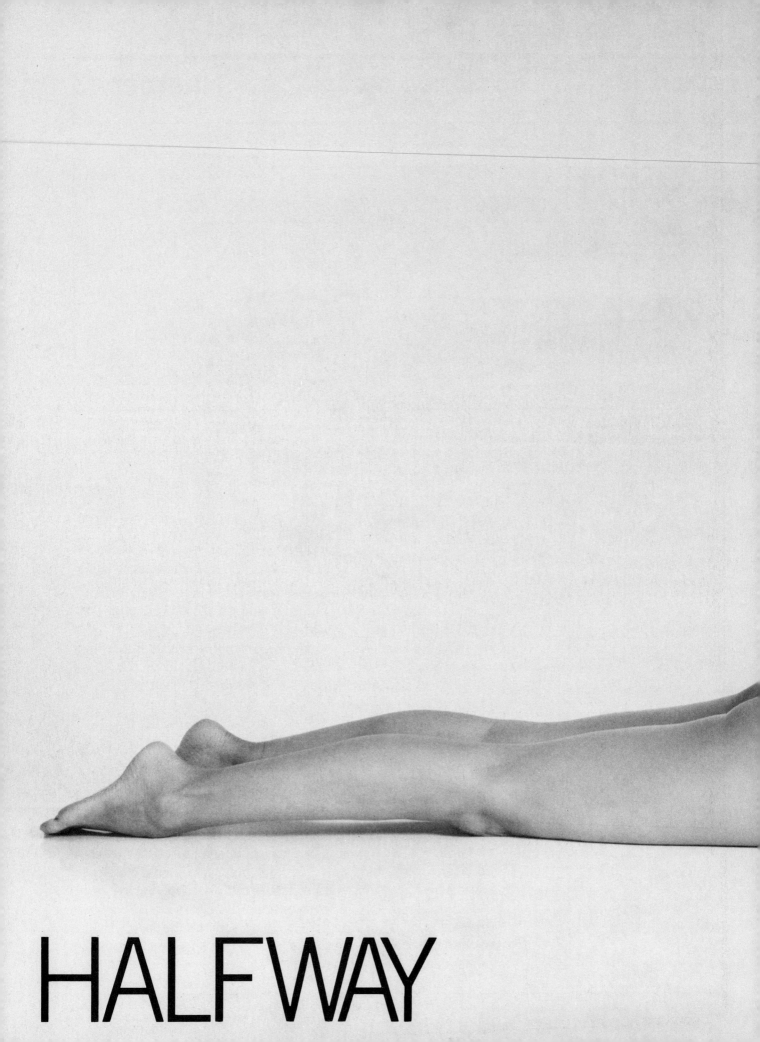

HALFWAY

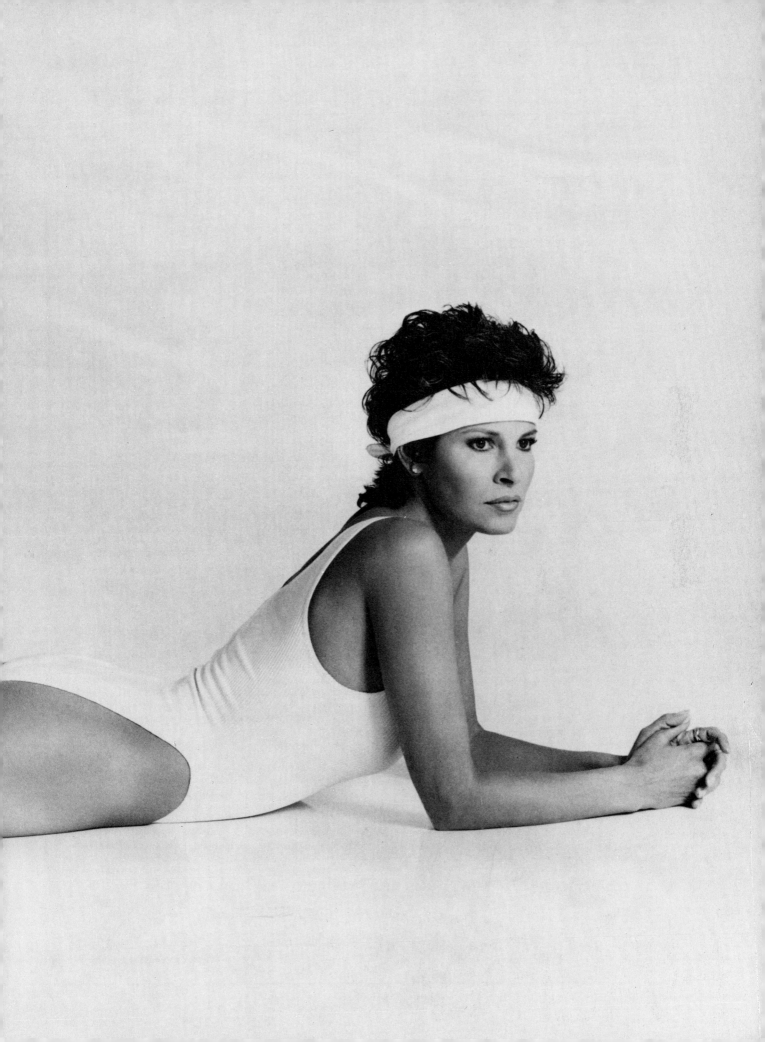

Halfway

Bravo! You made it this far. You deserve a hug, a kiss, a word of praise! But don't get too self-satisfied, because you're only halfway there.

This is an appropriate time to reveal that the Standing Postures you've just finished are basically warming-up exercises for beginners—the Floor Poses are the real physical stuff! They may give the appearance of being less so, but you'll still have to lie down to recover between each one of them.

Once you've mastered the opening series, you'll realize as much for yourself. You have just carefully laid out the framework for what's to come and can now apply those principles to practice.

Let's first review:

1. Breathing—for body rhythm and momentum.

2. Stretching—for mobility, circulation and stimulation.

3. Concentration—for direction and resolve.

4. Balance—for staying power, steadiness and centering.

5. Coordination—for combining and synchronizing.

6. Determination—for willpower.

7. Relaxation—to revitalize and de-stress.

8. Strength—to give structure and support.

9. Transition—to bridge the gaps smoothly.

10. Patience—for consistency and continuity.

11. Centering—to locate your base of power.

12. Stillness—to let it be.

Looking Ahead

In the sequence ahead, you'll be exercising muscles—mainly in your back—that have been neglected to a point of near apathy. So when you call them into use, they may not respond too readily. In such instances, *visualizing yourself mentally* in the finished pose comes in very handy. Try it: it's a sort of "mind over matter" approach or using the power of suggestion to stimulate your muscles when your normal reflexes fail.

Passive Aerobics

Below: *Animals are natural yogis—and my dobie is always an interested bystander at my morning sessions. She can't wait.*

From now on, the rest periods will be measured to 20 seconds, long enough to help you assimilate the benefits of each pose, but also short enough to keep up the flow of your aerobic activity. This way, you will not lose momentum and you will be able to build your stamina.

Enough said, shall we continue with the Floor Postures?

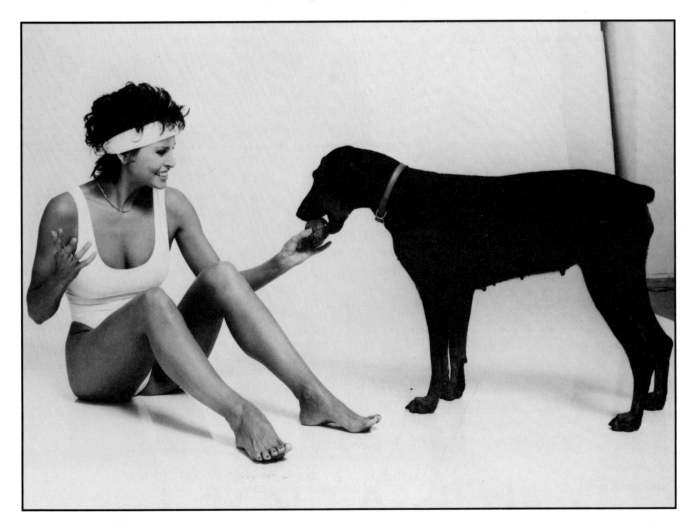

The Knee Squeeze

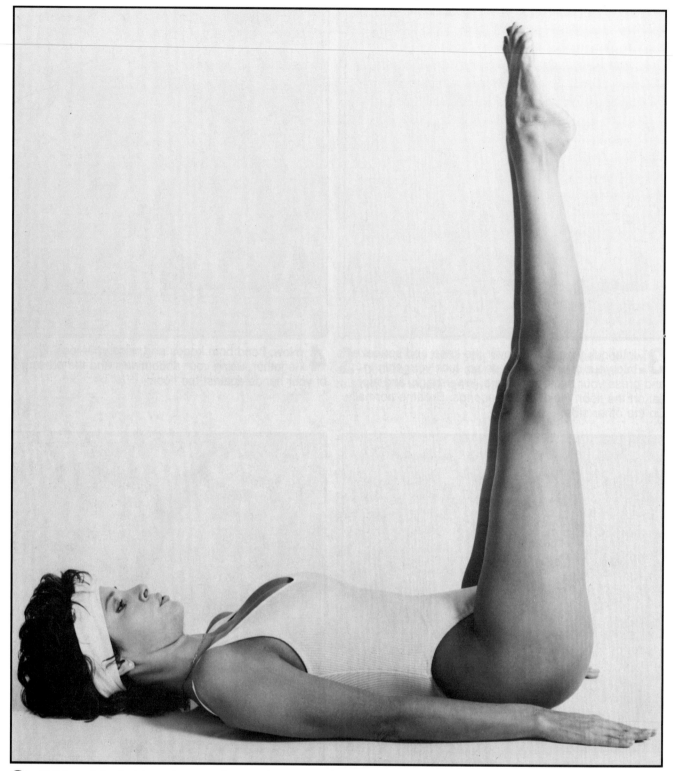

9. At this point, start lowering your legs, using the strength of your stomach muscles and the pressure of your arms and hands against the floor.

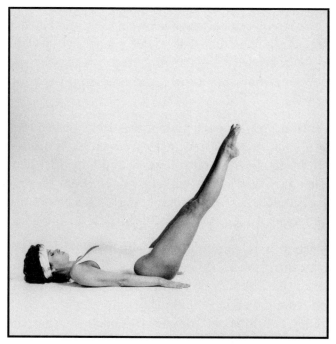

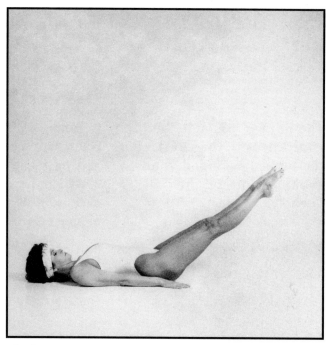

10. Keep lowering your legs slowly, with control. People with lower-back problems should put their hands under the buttocks and press down against the floor with their palms, to take the strain off the lower back.

11. Continue to lower the legs, keeping them completely straight, knees locked and toes pointed.

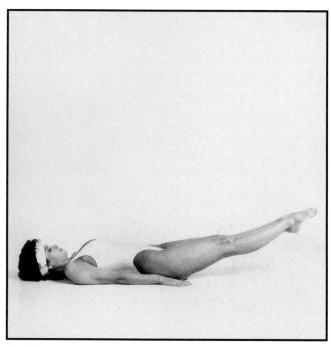

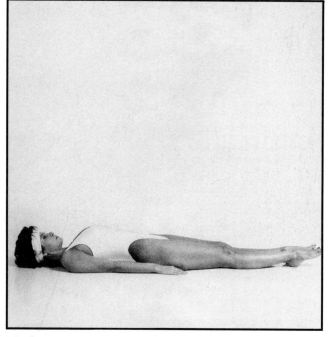

12. When you reach a point 6 to 12 inches off the floor, or wherever you feel the most abdominal tension, hold your legs there for 10 counts. Breathe normally.

13. Finally, lower your feet to the floor and relax. REPEAT the entire sequence, holding each section 20 counts. Rest.

The Knee Squeeze

Extra Help

The harder you squeeze your knees to the chest, the better, provided your shoulders are on the floor.

1. Coordinate. This pose coordinates the contraction and release in the spine and hip joints. The object is to get every inch of your spine to touch the floor, by tucking in your chin, pressing down with the abdomen, squeezing your knees, and releasing the hips. There's a lot going on!

2. Squeeze. The harder you squeeze your knees to the chest, the better, provided your shoulders are on the floor. If you have trouble getting a grip on your elbows over both legs, widen your grip, but don't let the pressure on your knees go. Try to get them to your chest even if your grip isn't perfect. On the single-knee pulls, remember to relax the opposite leg; try to keep the calf on the floor.

3. Lower. When you finish your double-leg squeeze, lower the legs back down with control; work those abdominals. Don't let your legs flop back down to the floor. Everything counts in this routine. If you have suffered from lower-back strain, I recommend that you put your hands under the hips, to support the back against the pull of the legs during the lowering.

4. Alternate Grip. For those who can squeeze the knees into the chest easily, try the elbow grip for the single-leg pulls as well. Just so you don't get lazy.

Words of Encouragement

This is not an also-ran pose . . . give it your all. While on your back, you are conditioning the spine for the postures ahead, so put your back into it.

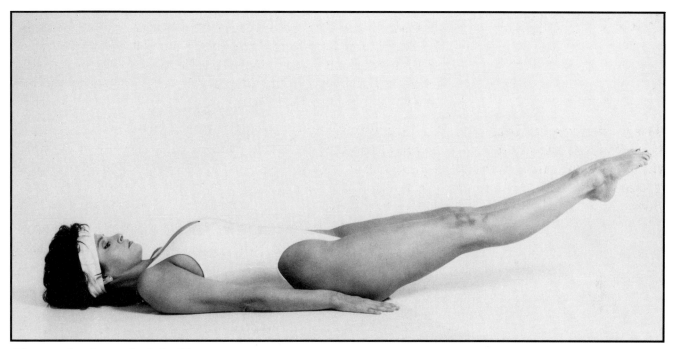

Above: *At the end of the Knee Squeeze, you may insert extra leg raises to work the lower abdomen. Just raise and lower your legs, without letting them touch the floor, 10–20 times.*

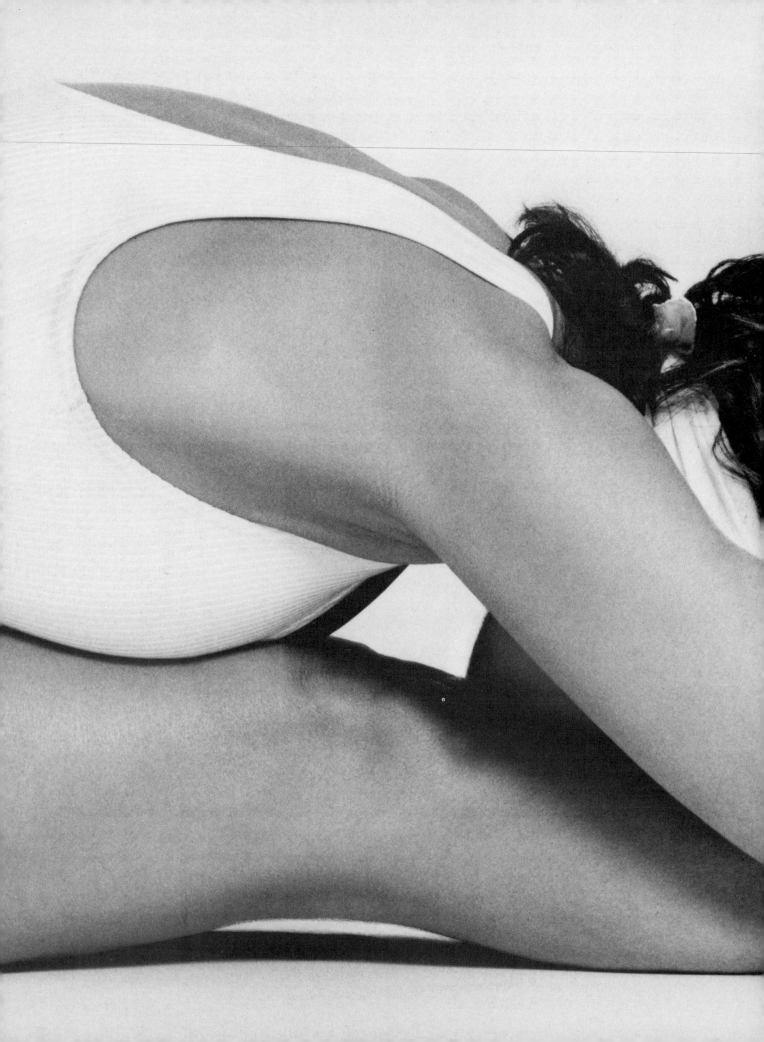

VITALITY

Swing-Up

This is probably the easiest version of a familiar friend, the sit-up, that anyone is ever likely to see.

The Swing-Up, along with the Dead Man's Pose, will be interlaced often through the ensuing floor postures. Let's get it right, so you can use it to revitalize yourself and to limber up progressively for the extreme stretches at the end of the routine.

This is probably the easiest version of a familiar friend, the sit-up, that anyone is ever likely to see. So if you follow the instructions exactly, you can really concentrate on what you're doing, with no excuses of cramping or strain.

Sit-ups can be problematical because they often put a strain on the back. But with the help of the arm swing, there's not much chance that your back will feel the pressure. However, if you can afford to do a more strenuous type of abdominal exercise, refer to the Extra Help section, paragraph 3, for ideas on how to fit them into this routine.

Benefits

- Firms and tightens the abdominal muscles. Slims the waistline.
- Stretches and works the hamstrings and the calves.
- Tones and stimulates abdominal organs.
- Improves digestion.

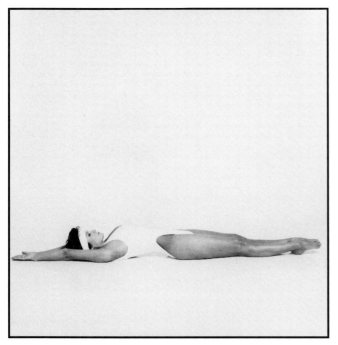

1. Lie flat on your back with your arms stretched over your head and with your legs tight, toes pointed. Your hands should be placed one on top of the other.

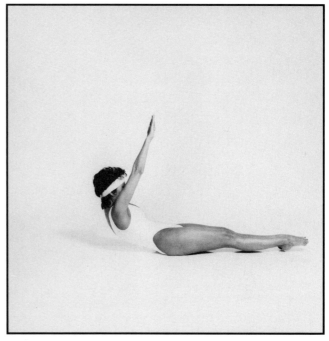

2. Inhale and, using your stomach muscles, swing your arms forward and sit up at the same time.

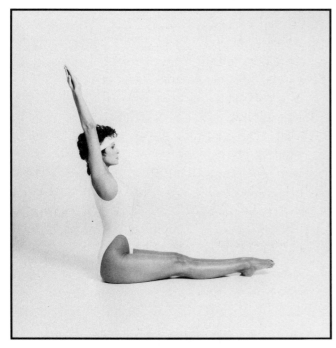

3. Once up, don't stop. Use the momentum of the swing to keep going over the legs.

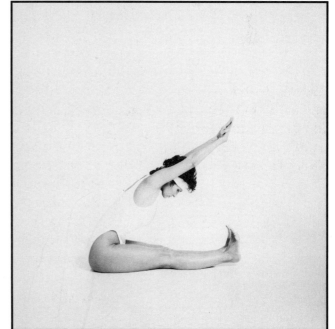

4. This is a very swift continuous movement. As you swing as far out over the legs as possible, flex your feet.

Swing-Up

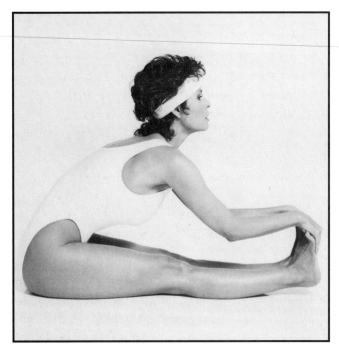

5. Grab hold of your feet with both hands and pull your toes toward you. If you can't reach your toes, take hold of your calves or ankles and pull until you feel a stretch in the back of the legs.

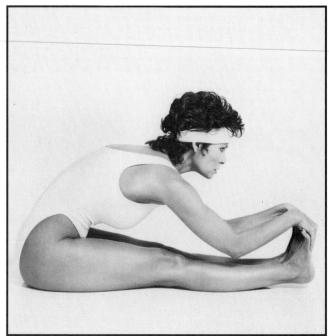

6. Inhale and scoot your hips out the back. Shimmy them backward while stretching up and over with your body. Keep the pull on your feet and, if possible, lift your heels off the floor.

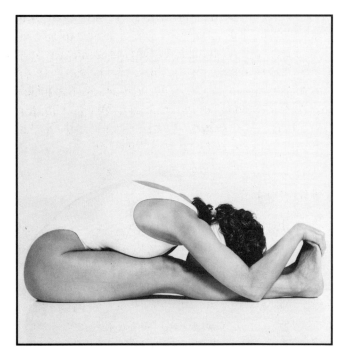

7. Now, pull yourself farther forward, bending your elbows downward. Stretch! Reach across your legs and put your stomach on your thighs.

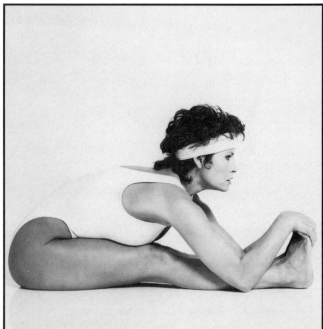

8. Exhale twice and drop your head to the legs. Now, that's a stretch! *Do it between each of the upcoming poses* when you are required to rest on your back. This is a good preparation for the Full Stretch later.

Extra Help

1. Swing. You can actually do the entire Swing-Up and stretch in one single motion once you become more limber. Just *swing* right over the legs, your momentum will carry you. Besides, you're warmed up now and should be able to do a snappy Swing-Up. I always exhale twice and give an extra pull at the very end for the stretch. Remember, these Swing-Ups are a preparation for the final super Full Stretch toward the end.

2. Hands to Feet. If you cannot reach your toes, grab hold of your ankles or calves and pull yourself forward. Flex your feet back toward you and try to get both heels off the ground. Also remember to scoot your bottom out behind you, to give a good stretch down the back of the legs.

3. Repetitions. When you want to work more on your abdominal muscles, do extra sets of the Swing-Up. This is the ideal point to insert them into the routine. You may also change your arm position to a favorite sit-up of your own, such as behind the head, crossed over the chest, or separated with palms turned up and knees bent. But whatever kind of abdominals you do, *finish with* one Swing-Up *exactly as described here.*

4. Leg Raises. While we're on the subject, to give extra work to the *lower* abdominals, you may add a set of leg raises while you are lowering the legs in the preceding posture. Use exactly the same body and arm position as on pages 128–29 and just raise and lower the legs in repetitions without letting them touch the ground. Do 10 or more. Remember that if you have lower-back or hip problems, it's very helpful to place your hands, palms down, just under your hips while you do any leg raises. It keeps the pull in the stomach, where it should be, and not on the lower back.

Words of Encouragement

Now you're ready to start the next cycle of postures, which works on the strengthening of the back. First the upper, the lower, then the whole spine, and finally arching the back like a wheel.

If you feel a momentary slump, that won't last. So press on. These upcoming poses will work your back in a way no other program or yoga method offers, a way that is distinctive to this routine. The sequence is certainly effective and invigorating, so look forward with enthusiasm!

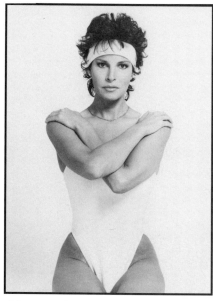

Above: *One alternate arm position for added abdominals.*

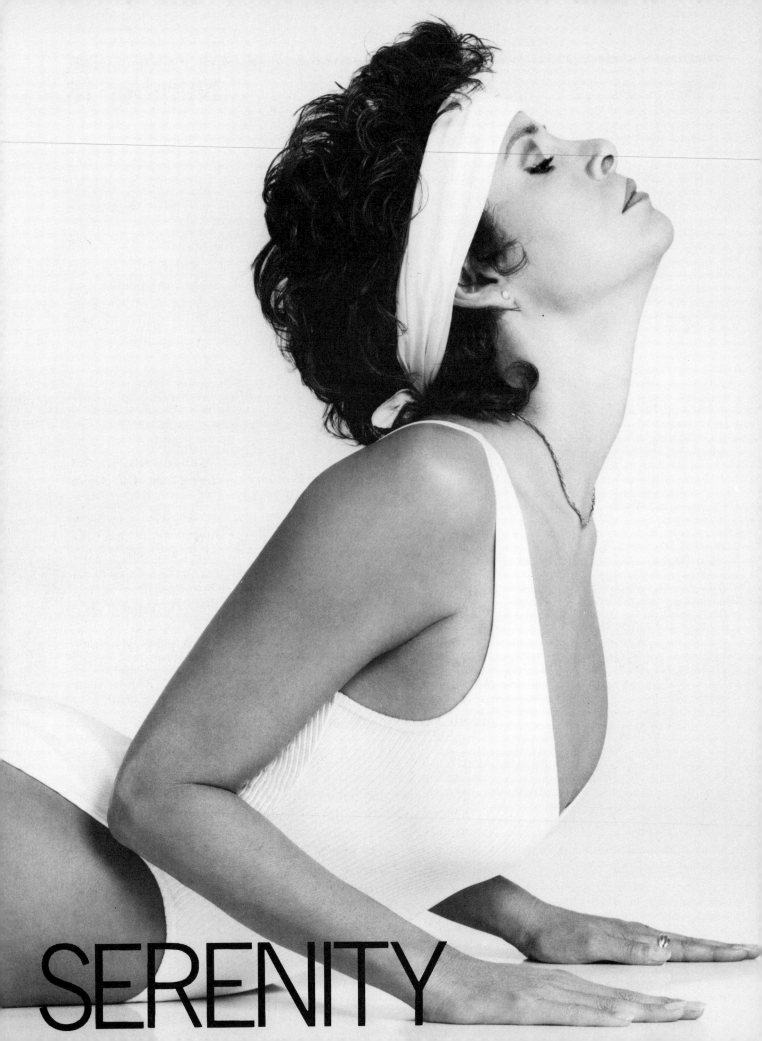

SERENITY

The Cobra

It can be a pretty humbling experience to realize that contact with the core of your vital energies is nearly nonexistent.

This is a classic, as perfect as a sphinx and as good for your health as any one thing you could possibly choose to do. But it also requires the mythic statue's serene resolve.

This is your first attempt to make contact with your all-important spine, and to use your spine strength alone to do the posture. Before, it came into play in connection with other parts of the body, but now it's almost entirely on its own. It may bring you down a notch or two, trying in vain to lift yourself up off the floor. It can be a pretty humbling experience to realize that contact with the core of your vital energies is nearly nonexistent.

This unimposing posture is not a shoo-in; the simplicity of it does not mean it's simple. In fact, simplicity in all things is the hardest to achieve. I know that I was doing the very impressive Bow and Standing Head to Knee postures long before I could hold the Cobra pose for a lousy 10 seconds.

Benefits

- Builds strength, limbers and increases the flexibility of the entire spine, from the lower back to the neck, vertebra by vertebra.
- Stretches and tones the muscles of the feet, legs, abdomen, chest, back, and neck.
- Stimulates the abdominal organs, especially the intestines, liver, stomach, and spleen.
- Helps relieve menstrual irregularities and pains.
- Helps correct and cure spinal disorders such as lumbago, slipped disc, rheumatism, lower backaches, etc.

The Cobra

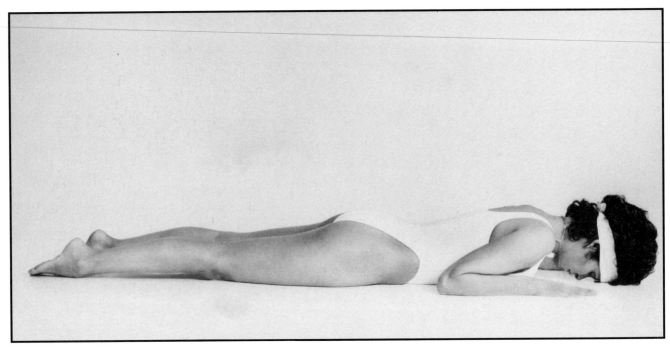

1. From the Swing-Up, roll over on your stomach and face the floor. Your head should face the mirror. Place your hands, face-down, under your shoulders, near the breasts.

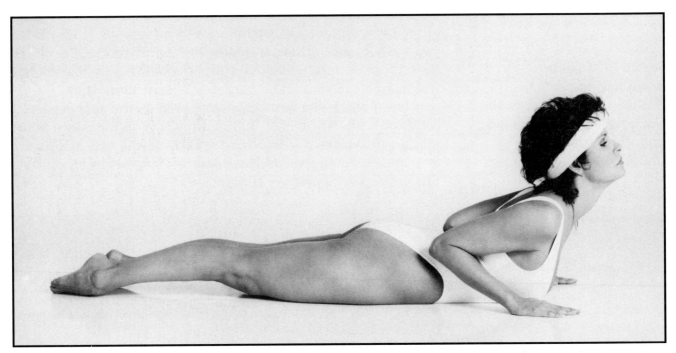

3. Inhale and slowly lift your upper body, head back and hands pressing against the floor. As you arch back, don't straighten your arms all the way.

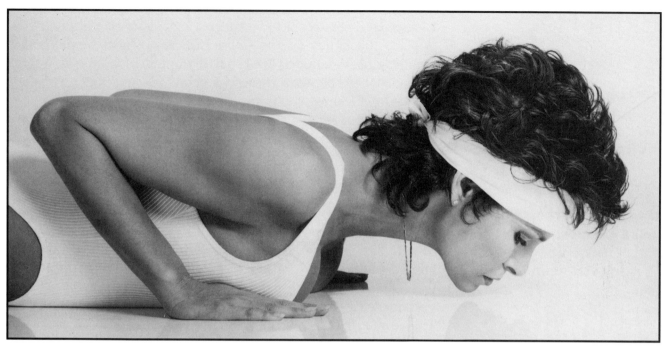

2. Place your chin on the floor. Where exactly you place your hands depends on your proportions. For some, it's next to the breasts; for others, it's at shoulder level. See Extra Help.

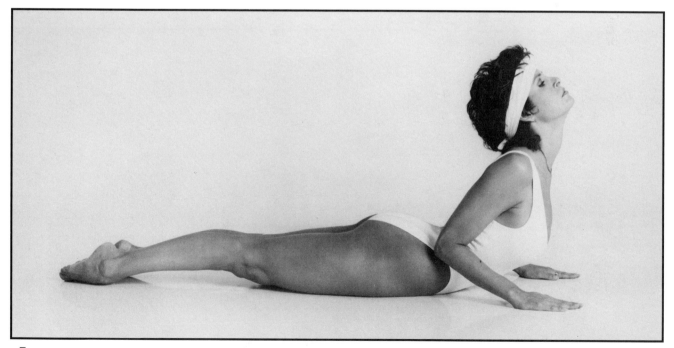

4. Exhale and keep lifting until your upper body is arched off the floor from your navel to your head. Drop your head still farther back, keeping your elbows close to your sides. Your arms should form a 90-degree angle at the elbow. Hold the position for 20 seconds, breathing normally. Lower yourself to the floor. Rest *20 seconds* on your stomach—head to the side. REPEAT.

The Cobra

Extra Help

It's very important to make an effort calmly and consistently, without showing strain on the face.

Below: *Treat the rest period between each of the floor postures as a short moment of blissful relaxation. But don't doze off, keep those eyes open and your mind in the present.*

1. Hands. There seem to be various schools of thought on where to place the hands for the Cobra. Some say next to the breast, some say past shoulder level, but if the truth be known, I think it's somewhere between these two points, depending on your proportions. Of course, you'll have to use your arms to get you up in the Cobra, but after a week or so rely less and less on them and rely more on your back and buttock muscles.

2. Elbows. The object is to bend the elbows so that they are at *right angles* and point them into your sides to keep the strength centered in the back and not on the arms.

3. The Head. The head should go back, eyes looking up, mouth closed, face calm without grimacing. It's very important to make an effort calmly and consistently, without showing strain on the face. Direct your effort to the correct point—in this case, the lower-back muscles—and don't let it run all over and settle on your face. This idea will keep you from overstraining; get it out of your mind that you can do this any old way—you have to be precise and use control.

4. Shoulders. The shoulders do have a tendency to ride up, so consciously think about keeping them down. The elbows pointing to the waist help this to some extent.

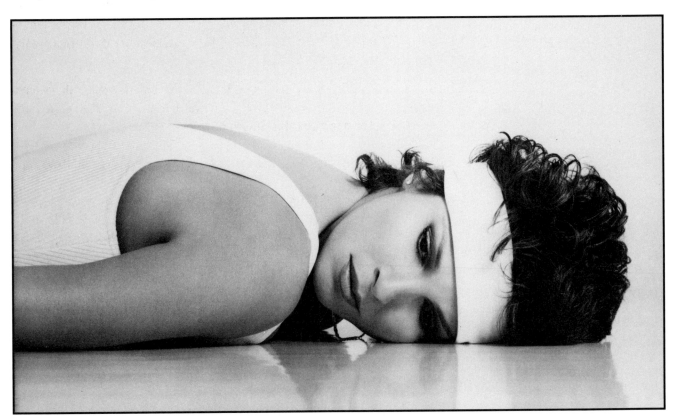

5. Staying. Staying in this pose is not so simple the first times you try it. After all, you are probably using your back in a way that you've never experienced before. It may all seem strangely numb back there and you feel somewhat like a beached whale. That only proves how much you need this. And that's what's going to change. You are going to become familiar with all your back muscles and learn how to use them.

6. Legs. The legs should be straight together and tight throughout, the toes pointed. Before you even start the pose, check their position and tighten the buttocks. Then inhale and begin.

7. Breathing. Begin to come up on your inhale. Then exhale and breathe normally. In the early stages this pose can take more energy than you expect so don't hold your breath—that creates tension on the face, to say nothing of the fact that it totally inhibits you.

8. Arch. When you arch your upper body back, keep the navel touching the floor and don't come all the way up. You'll have a chance before long to arch back fully, but take it gradually step by step. For now press your navel to the floor.

9. Charley Horse. Lots of people get kinks or cramps in their legs when they first start. I did and if I'm out of practice, I still do. But just flex your feet to get rid of them and move on. If they persist, as they sometimes do, don't give it too much importance. Struggle on. The kinks and charley horses will disappear with regular practice.

10. Rest. During each rest period in this and the next three postures, alternate the side that your head rests on. This way, both sides of your neck get equal time.

Words of Encouragement

I never particularly enjoyed this business of lying face-down on a towel with only the terry-cloth piles to contemplate. The only reason I stuck to it at first was I got ticked off that I couldn't raise my nose off the floor more than a few inches. I hated this feeling of helplessness and decided I'd have to lick it. My commitment paid off—it will for you, too. So when you find yourself in that position and hating it, think of me . . . you can lick it, too.

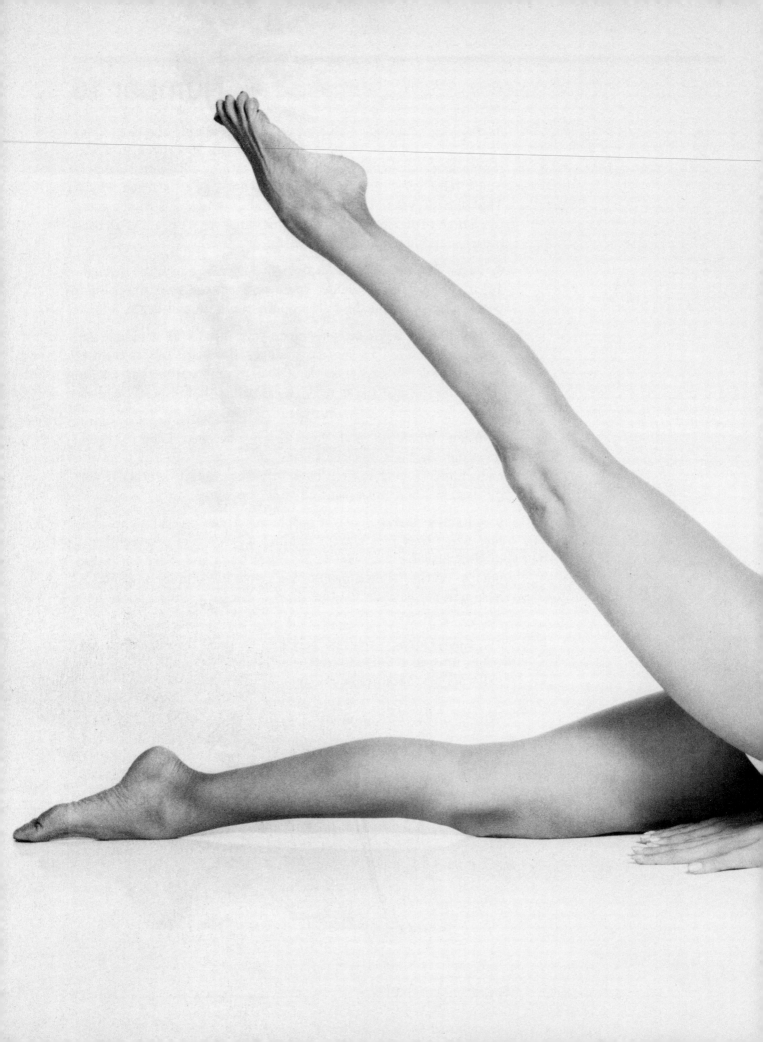

FAITH

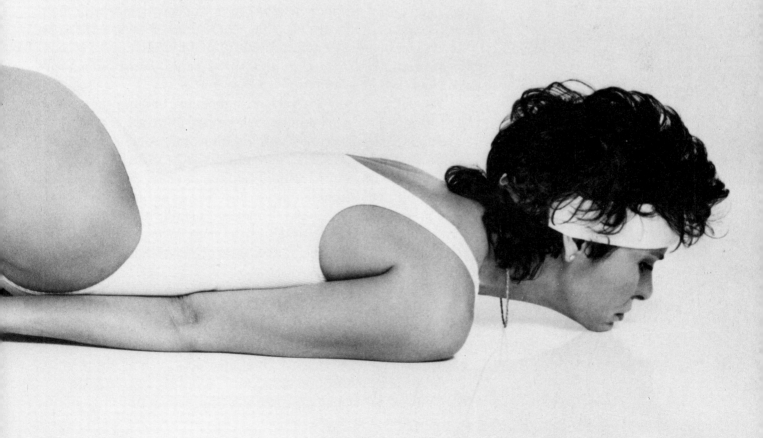

The Locust

T he approach to this pose is not easy to pinpoint. In the beginning it seems akin to blind effort; first, because you can't see yourself in the posture (your head is too low or facing down throughout). You almost always feel that you're doing less well than you
are; and since any attempt to check yourself in the mirror is coun-
terproductive, your faith in yourself is being tested, along with
your patience and resolve.

Secondly, you can't tell what's happening because the muscle-
to-brain signals of the lower spine are rusty from lack of use. You'll
have to develop new connections with different resources, and you'll
be pleasantly surprised at how effective they can be. Initially,
you'll have to rely on reaching into the numbness and rummaging
around until you stumble upon a clue. But, eventually, something
more precise shines through. This point usually crystallizes when
you begin to *visualize* yourself in the pose. What you see is what
you'll get . . . it's simply using the power of suggestion. And it works!

Benefits

- Strengthens and stretches the lower-back area and the legs.
- Tightens and firms the hips and buttocks.
- Helps cure and prevent spinal disorders such as slipped disc,
  lower-back pains, and sciatica.
- Tones the abdomen, stimulates the abdominal organs, and
  improves digestion.
- Increases the pulse rate.

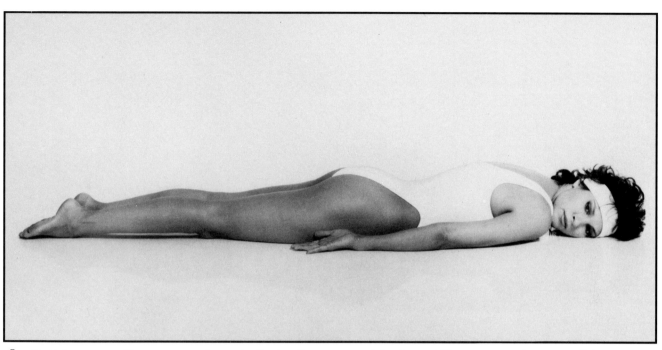

1. Start from a position on your stomach. During the course of the Locust Pose, your pulse rate will increase significantly. So, concentrate on breathing normally. *Do not hold your breath!*

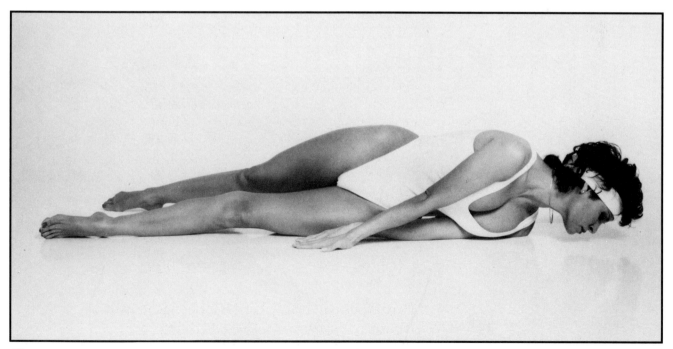

2. Roll your body back on one side and place one hand underneath your thighs, then roll to the other side and place the other hand next to it. The palms should be face-down on the floor. Your little fingers should be touching.

The Locust

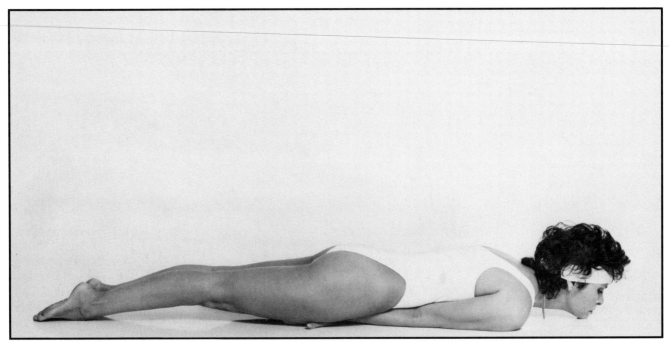

3. Roll your body back over on top of your arms and rest your chin on the floor. Spread your fingers beneath you. Keep the legs together, feet touching.

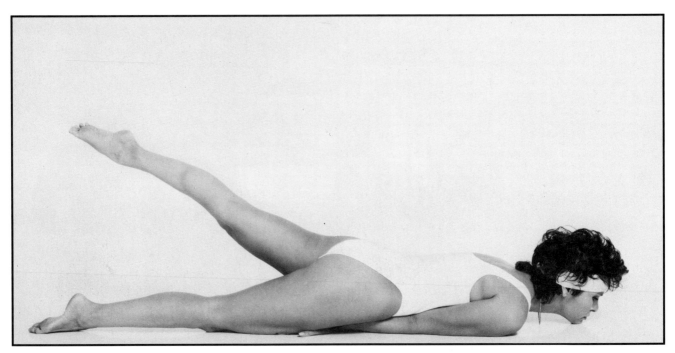

5. Do exactly the same thing with your left leg, making sure that your hip doesn't lift off the arm. Point back and up with your leg and hold it for 10 counts. Don't worry if one leg goes higher than the other! It's normal.

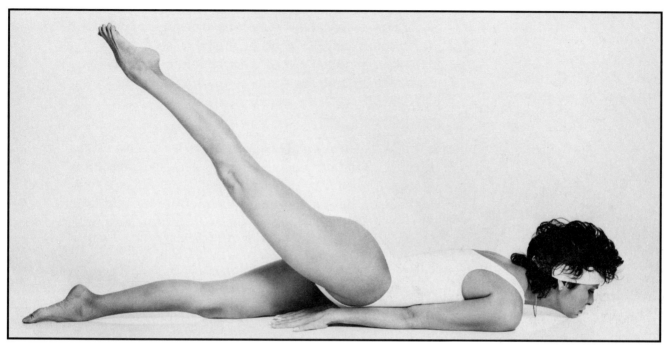

4. Inhale and, without raising your hip off the arm, lift your right leg straight back and up, toes pointed and knee locked. Hold your leg there for 10 counts. Breathe normally. Then, lower it back to the floor.

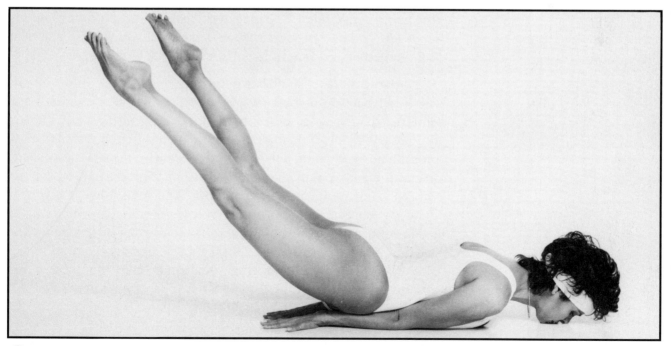

6. Next place your mouth on the floor. Take a deep breath, tighten the leg muscles and buttocks, and press your hands against the floor. On the exhale, bring both legs up! Hold for 10 full counts. Breathe normally. Lower your legs slowly, rest 20 seconds, and REPEAT.

The Locust

Extra Help

1. Hands and Arms. Placing the arms under the body seems like an awkward move at first, but after a few times you do it automatically. Just roll to one side, slide one arm under, roll to the other side, and do the same. If you have any difficulty, however, just refer back to the photos and captions to help sort out what goes where.

2. Face. The face on the floor in step 6 is somewhat disconcerting. But it's for the purpose of keeping your neck absolutely straight when you raise your legs up behind. Some schools teach the chin on the floor, but for beginners the mouth touching the floor gives extra leverage and I find it's easier to get the legs higher. And, of course, you'll be on a towel.

3. Beforehand. Before you lift both legs back, get your arms well situated under the body, spreading your fingers out beneath you. Then straighten your legs and tighten the buttocks. Now visualize what the pose looks like and get a clear picture of it in your mind. Inhale deeply and lift your legs into position on the exhalation. Since in the beginning you are unfamiliar with which muscles to use and how to coordinate them, visualizing can be an important tool.

4. The Lift. When you lift both legs together they may separate and point in a V. That's alright in the beginning, but after holding for a few counts try to bring the legs together, or at least close them together just before lowering them back down.

5. Aerobic Value. This pose definitely has aerobic value. It gets the heart beating faster and your cardiovascular system is stimulated strongly. A lot seems to be happening in the final stage of the pose. So your best approach is to remain calm, remember to breathe normally, and don't hold your breath. It's perfectly normal to sputter and puff in the early stages of your practice—even advanced students have their moments. You will be more aware of it in a quiet atmosphere than if you were being drowned out by loud music. So don't inhibit yourself—you're entitled to moan and groan a little to get things going. Don't be ashamed of making an all-out effort. You're attacking something new. It's good to feel absolutely ridiculous. Laugh at yourself. It never hurts.

Words of Encouragement

Below: *After this pose, I always feel like coming up for air. But don't be afraid of making an all-out effort. You're attacking something new. It's alright to feel absolutely ridiculous. Laugh at yourself. It never hurts.*

This is a challenge. Your resolve will be tested in the Locust. Just realize that's the game and play it. Every muscle may go into hysterics and your senses may seem overloaded. But let it happen, nothing bad will come of it. You are taking charge of your reflexes, maybe for the first time, and they are going into a mock revolt. Hold your ground. Monitor your breath, but don't "hold it." Follow it in and out—if you learn to trust it, it won't let you down. Find your center within the storm of bodily protests . . . and watch the revolt die.

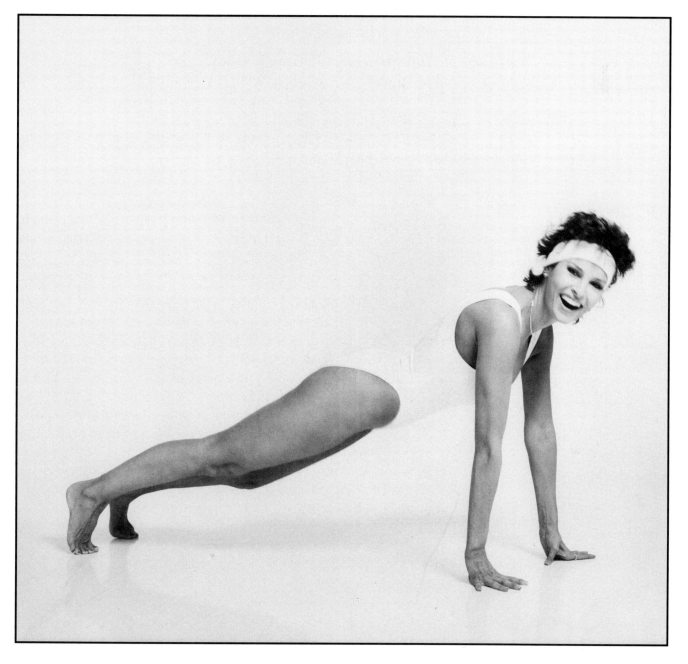

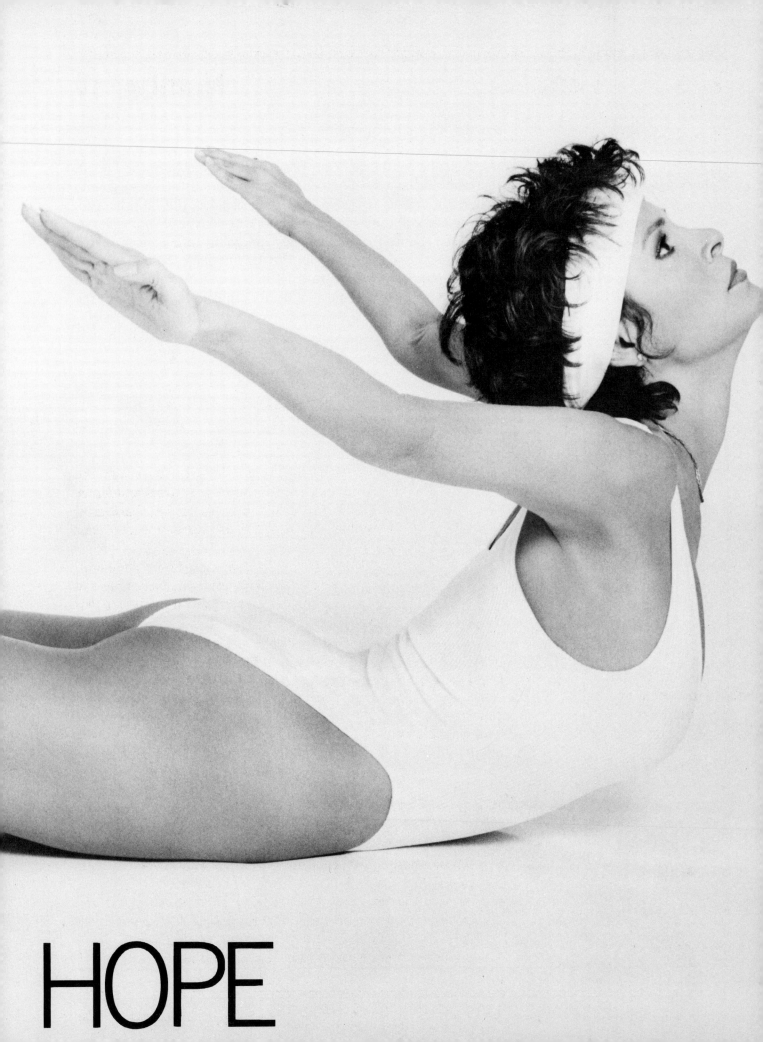

HOPE

Getting airborne is the first priority.

T his pose is very similar to the Locust—in fact, it's a sister. The difference is that, before, you had the use of your arms and hands to raise your legs up; here you must rely solely on your back muscles. That's why it's called *Full* Locust: because the support of your entire back comes into play.

As you are already aware, contact and control over these back muscles can be very elusive at first. So, once again, you'll have to help yourself by visualizing the position in your mind before getting into it.

As a beginner, it seems to be easier if you take mental flight instead of being grounded by trying to analyze what muscles do what. Later, after you're flying, you can make connections and refinements. Getting airborne is the first priority. No matter how you do on your first few tries, remain hopeful and optimistic. These qualities, although seldom mentioned in exercise programs, are often the ones that bring the best results—ask any physical therapist.

Benefits

- Tightens and firms the hips and buttocks.
- Stimulates, strengthens, and stretches the entire musculature.
- Specifically firms and limbers the front of the body, hip and shoulder joints, spine, neck, upper arms, chest, abdomen, pelvic area, and thighs.
- Increases the size and elasticity of the rib cage.

The Full Locust

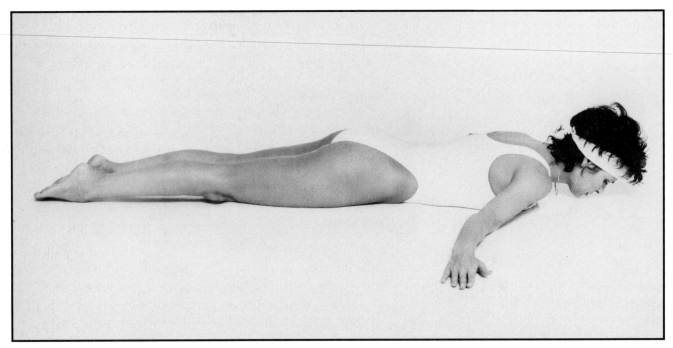

1. While you're lying on your stomach, bring your arms out to the sides at approximately shoulder level. Place your chin on the floor in front of you. Tighten the muscles of your legs and point your toes. Prepare to lift both arms and legs simultaneously.

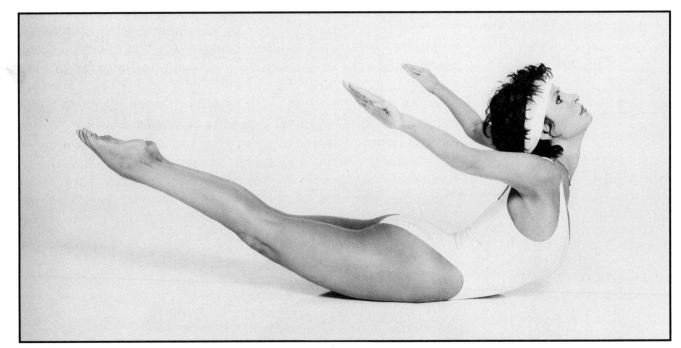

2. Inhale deeply. On your exhale, lift your arms and legs off the floor in a single fluid movement, using the strength of your upper and lower back. Stretch your arms to the back and sides and keep lifting them. Relax your shoulders and don't let them rise up. Hold for 10 seconds, breathing normally. Then come down smoothly, and relax for *20 seconds,* with your head to the side. REPEAT.

Extra Help

1. Tiredness. By this time you may experience a slump in your energy. That's because you're learning and it takes twice the amount of your resources to adapt yourself to something new. But pushing on will increase your stamina. And you'll find that you're completely revitalized by the end.

2. Trying. Sometimes doing the postures without trying too hard works wonders. It's no joke! I've found that, if I didn't get myself all psyched up to it, I could then do a posture I thought I couldn't. Sometimes the approach should be: I'll just do it and see what happens.

3. Lifting Off. This pose can be pretty frustrating in the learning stages. Especially when you try to lift off and nothing happens. The consolation is that a lot more is happening than you can imagine. Eventually you will be successful, but in the meantime don't give up—there's lots of work to do to re-establish your muscle reflexes. Tell yourself when you don't lift off that at least the ground crews are busy.

Tell yourself when you don't lift off that at least the ground crews are busy.

Words of Encouragement

This posture is great for the body, but it takes everything you've got to do it. It's the most difficult pose in the series for me. I finally had to resort to flights of fancy, as I lay there with my chin on the floor. I thought of my arms as wings and spread them to the side as if to fly. Then I took a deep breath and gave myself the mental lightness of gliding unperturbed over any difficulty; with this in mind, I was able to get my arms and legs into a good position to stay up there through the 10 counts. After a few weeks I grew to like it up there.

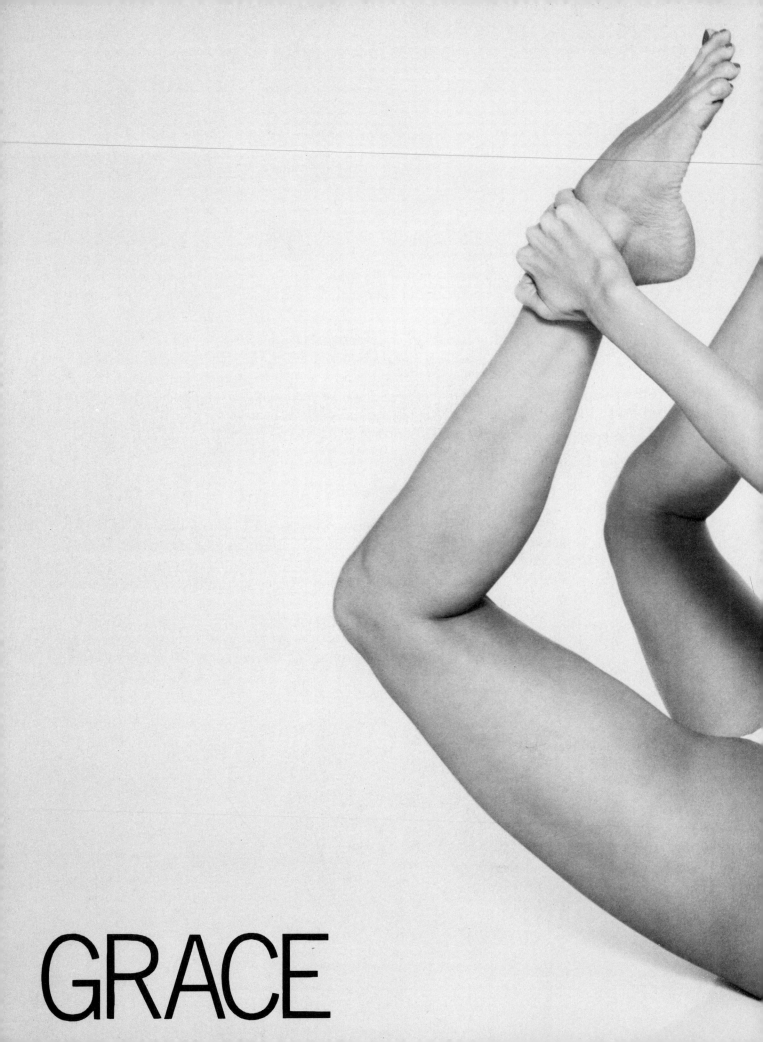

GRACE

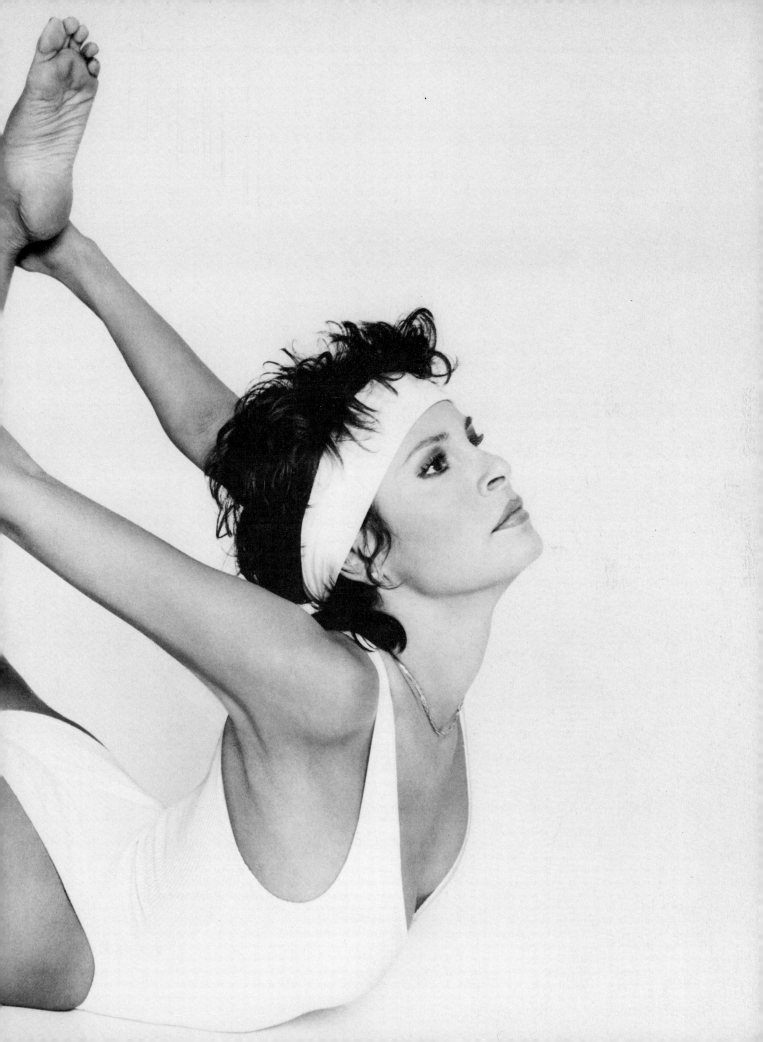

The Bow

The Bow Pose is the crowning effort of everything we've been working on through the last three postures, starting with the Cobra. There, we worked the upper torso; then the lower torso with the Locust; then the full torso with the Full Locust; and now the ultimate arch and lift of the full torso, with the Bow. It's a gradual process.

As I said before, these floor postures are particularly difficult, because of the remedial work needed on the back of your body to build your strength and flexibility and also to sharpen the connections between your brain, central nervous system, and muscles. So keep moving steadily in that direction. This is the last of the building blocks in this backward-lifting series, reinforcing your efforts and bringing you closer to your destination and the multiple benefits therein.

Benefits

- Combines the benefits of the Cobra, Locust and Full Locust poses.
- Improves the flexibility and maintains the elasticity of the entire spine, aligning each vertebra properly.
- Tightens and firms the muscles of the back, upper arms, abdomen, and thighs.
- Stretches and limbers shoulder, hip, and knee joints.

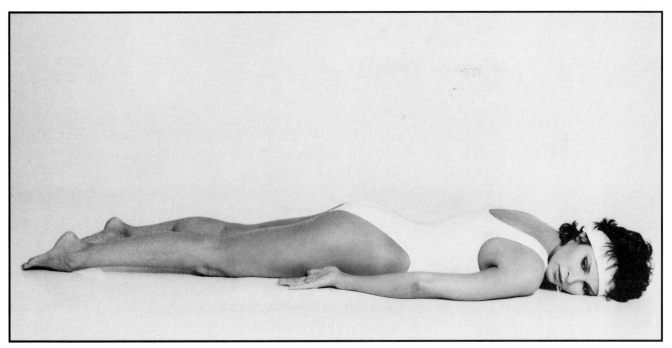

1. Keep your eyes open during your rest periods—it keeps your energy up—don't drowse. You may be breathing heavily from the effort of the last posture, so relax and feel yourself inhale and exhale involuntarily.

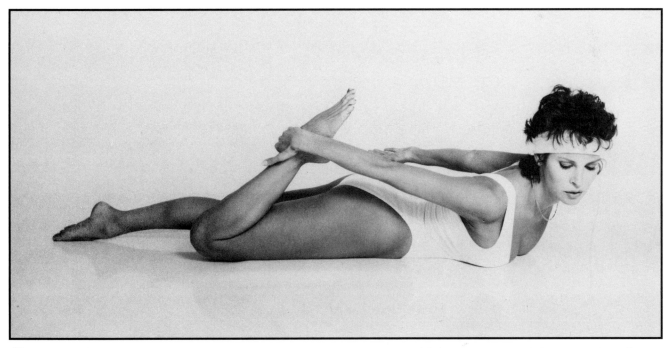

2. From the position on your stomach, reach around and take hold of first one ankle and then the other. The exact placement of the hand depends on your proportions. It is also acceptable to hold your feet.

The Bow

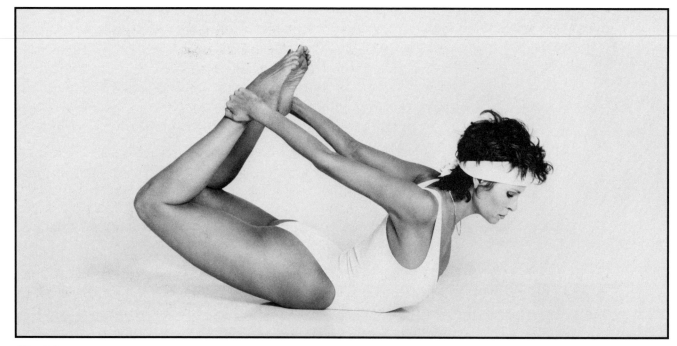

3. When you have hold of both ankles or feet, try keeping your knees no more than a foot apart. They like to spread, so keep a rein on them. Now, take a deep breath and on the exhale start lifting your chest and head up, while simultaneously kicking up and back with your legs.

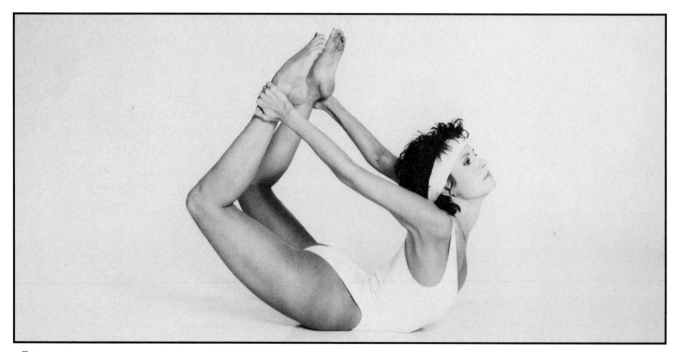

4. Keep kicking up higher, using your buttock muscles. Let your chest expand and pull with your arms. Stay up there for 20 seconds. Breathe normally. Lower yourself down slowly, rest 20 seconds on your stomach and REPEAT. Rest again for 20 seconds, eyes open, head to the side.

Extra Help

1. Holding the Feet. Some of you may have difficulty grabbing the feet behind you, or your knees may ache with the strain. Don't worry. It's natural that you may feel stiff in the beginning. So don't use that as an excuse for quitting. Even if you can just hold your feet and nothing else, you're going to reap benefits. If you need to open your knees wider in order to grasp the feet, do so.

2. Kicking Back. When raising the legs do not pull them back to your bottom. But lift them up and away from the body. If your kicking muscles are not strong enough, concentrate on using your buttock muscles and press your navel to the floor. This will serve to activate your muscles in that area, so that eventually you can bring them into play.

3. Knees. Try not to let the knees drift too far apart, but use your own common sense. If your legs won't go up very far without separating more, allow your knees to separate past the 12-inch maximum suggested.

4. Rock Forward. When your legs are in your best position, rock forward slightly and kick up. This movement usually makes it easier for the legs to go higher.

5. Cramping. Here come those cramps again! Think nothing of it. It's very common for beginners. Treat them as you would a fly at a picnic—a nuisance but nothing serious.

Words of Encouragement

Do you feel somewhat like a turtle that's been turned helplessly over on its back?

Do you feel somewhat like a turtle that's been helplessly over on its back? Understandable, but soon you'll be arching gracefully back and feeling the exact opposite of awkward.

This is not an especially hard posture for most people. But it does take some getting used to. It may not be love at first sight, but it grows on you!

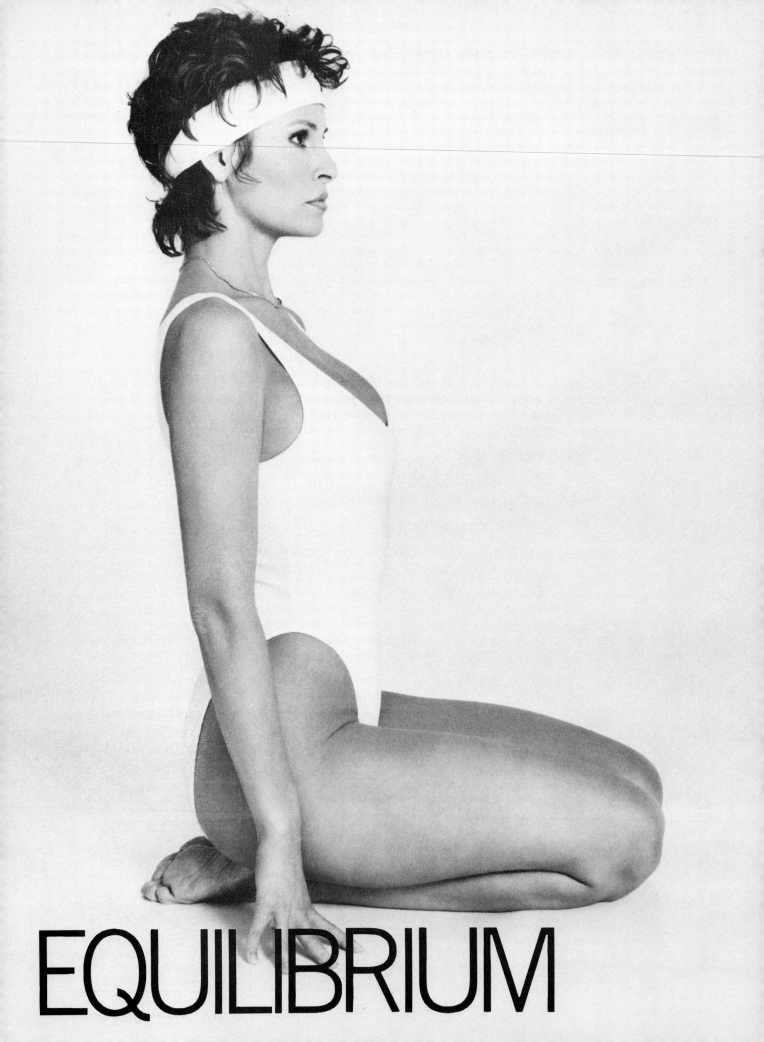

EQUILIBRIUM

This is a perfect pose to realign the body after the last few postures, which concentrated so specifically on the back muscles. It is the ideal way to equalize and adjust the different forces and energies in the body. And that is what equilibrium—mental or physical—is all about: a total state of balance between you and the world.

Benefits

- Fully extends, stretches, and works the dorsal (back) region, lower back, abdomen, thighs, knees, calves, and ankles.
- Helps relieve and prevent lower backaches, sciatica, and rheumatisms of the legs.

The Kneeling Pose

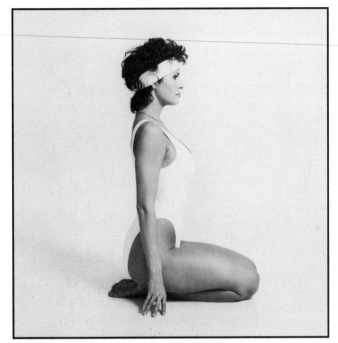

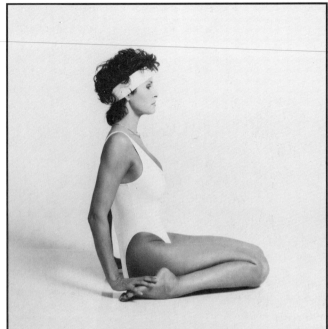

1. Start by sitting on your heels, knees together, arms at your sides, back straight.

2. Open the feet and allow your hips to rest on the floor between them. Place your hands on your feet. If you cannot keep your knees together, let them open slightly to accommodate your hips on the floor.

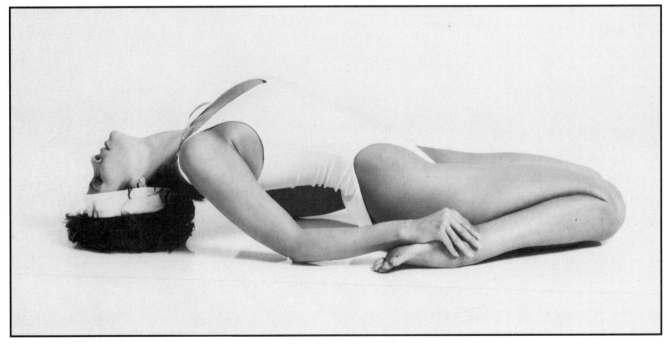

5. Keep lowering your head backward farther and farther until it rests on the floor. Support yourself all the way with your arms, allowing your back to arch as well.

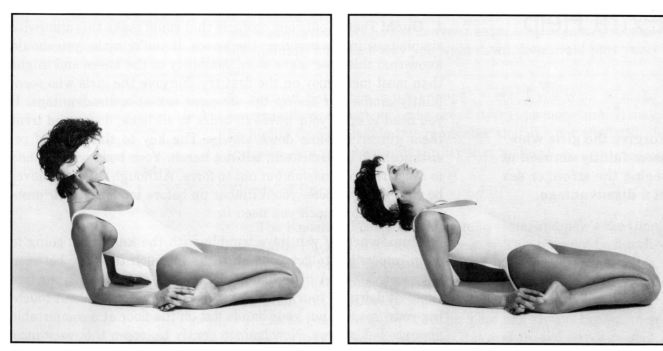

3. Now, lower yourself back, first on one elbow, then the other. Prepare to drop your head backward.

4. Now, supporting yourself on your bent arms, drop your head back.

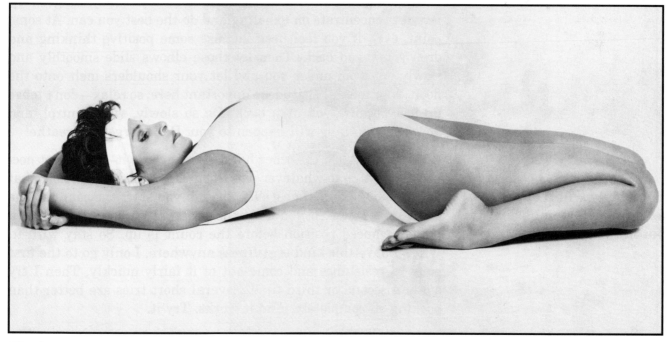

6. Slowly ease your shoulders onto the floor and curl your head forward until the back of your neck touches the floor also. Lastly, bring your arms behind your head and grasp the opposite elbows. Stay there for 20 seconds, pressing the knees together. Breathe normally. Come up the same way you went down. Rest for 20 seconds on your back, swing up, and REPEAT.

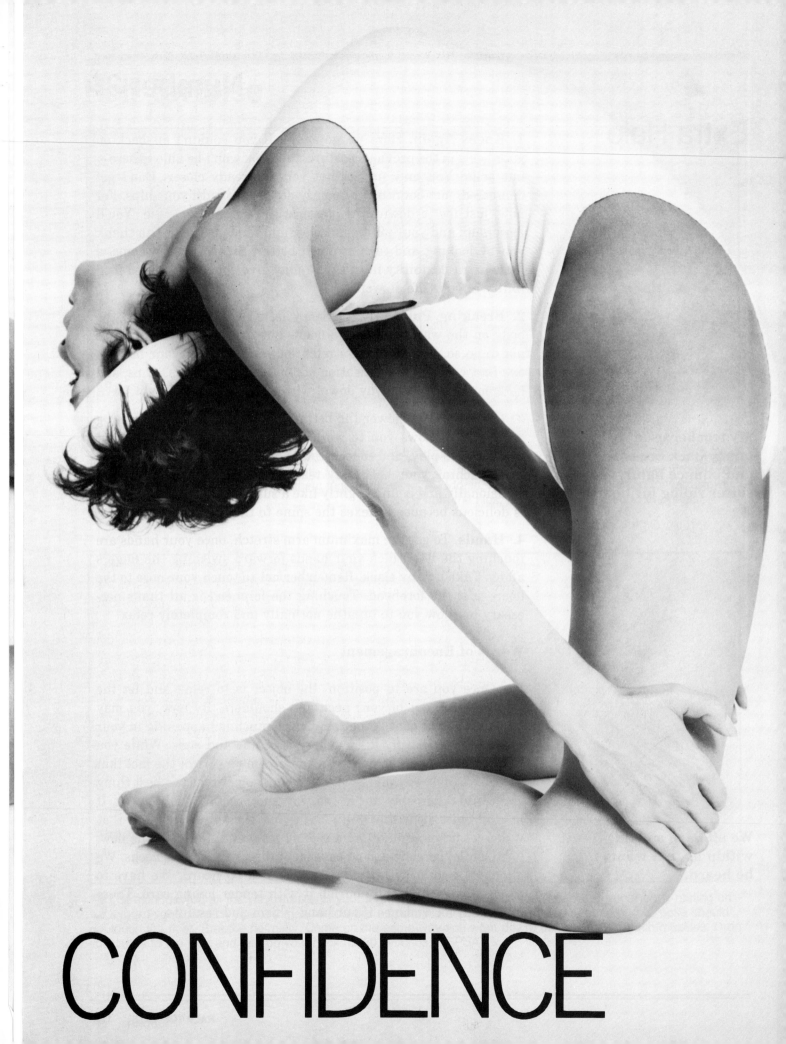

CONFIDENCE

I found that this pose builds enormous confidence when done slowly and with relaxed breathing. It seems to break down the fear of bending backward, which is quite common and natural but inhibits us from using our body fully.

When we realize we have more latitude than we think, we are rewarded not only by physical benefits but also with newfound confidence in our ability to overcome obstacles and the fear that goes with them. I had to work into this posture gradually, but it had a very exhilarating effect when accomplished and held. It also helped my stamina and my breath control for singing.

Benefits

- Builds flexibility and tones the entire spine, from the lower back to the neck.
- Fully stretches and tones the front of the body, including the abdominal organs, the chest, and the glands located in the throat such as the thyroid and the parathyroid.
- Firms and slims the waistline, abdomen, and legs.
- Corrects drooping rounded shoulders, expands the chest, and relieves backaches.
- Activates blood circulation in the spinal nervous system.

The Camel

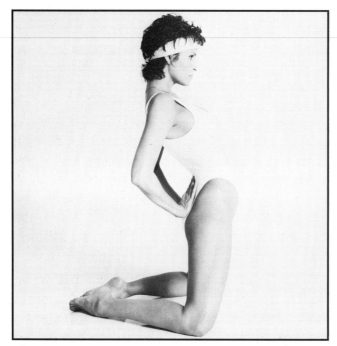

1. Position yourself on your knees, feet not more than 8 inches apart, knees a little wider. Keep your hips square to the front, and place your hands on your hips or lower back, heels down, fingers up.

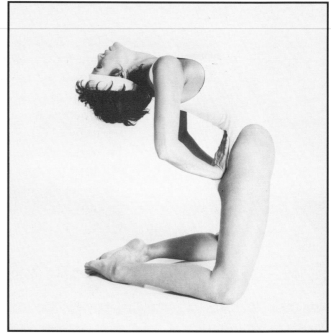

2. Now, drop your head on an exhale, arching back as far as possible. Use your arms on the hips to support yourself. You will not fall. Breathe normally.

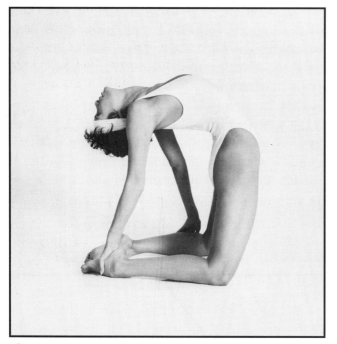

3. Slowly reach down with one hand and take hold of your upturned foot. Then do the other side. Place your palms on the heels, your fingers on the inside, thumbs outside, arching back as you do so.

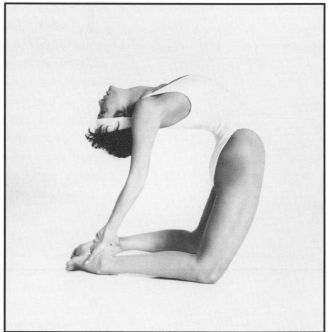

4. Grip your heels *firmly,* pressing your hips and pelvis slowly forward. Feel the stretch along the front of your thighs. Hold for 20 seconds. *Come up very slowly,* using your hands on the hips for support. Rest for 20 seconds on your back. REPEAT.

Extra Help

As Franklin Delano
Roosevelt once said,
"The only thing we have
to fear is fear itself."

1. Fear of Falling. If you follow the step-by-step description under the photos, it will serve you well. There is everything there you'll need except, of course, your mental approach. Many people are afraid of bending backward, because they have an inbred fear of falling that inhibits them. But in this posture you couldn't have more safeguards, especially if you work *slowly*. You have your hands first on the hips, then on the feet, to support your every move. What you must build on your own is confidence in your ability to do it! Your body is ready, willing, and able. Not to be melodramatic, but as Franklin Delano Roosevelt once said, "The only thing we have to fear is fear itself." And truer words were never spoken. Don't let your fear inhibit you from doing your best in this posture and in life.

2. Exhalation. Exhalation and relaxation are your allies in your fight to break down the tension that comes with fear. A measure of patience also helps. Breathe through the points of tension as you come to them, especially in the small of the back. Give yourself a chance to get through barriers that have built up over a long time. After all, you are doing movements that are unfamiliar to you.

3. Small of the Back. Press your hips forward, feel the grace of the movement ever so subtly in your spine, and go with the flow. Ironically enough, if you are the limber type you must use some caution because the final position you achieve is more extreme. Those who have to fight rigidity should not worry. Just keep arching back against resistance; you'll feel great when it's over.

4. Coming Up. Come up slow, slow, slow. You may feel a little tipsy, so lie down and let yourself equalize for 20 seconds.

Words of Encouragement

Your body is your friend: use it and trust it, explore its many resources, and have faith in yourself. Leave the anxiety on the sidelines, even for just a brief moment, and you'll prove to yourself that you had the confidence all along. It was just hiding behind a thin veneer of fear. So call its bluff.

The Advanced Camel

This is an advanced version of the Camel which is offered for those of you who are very limber. You may wish to include it as the second set. However, it is optional and not recommended for beginners.

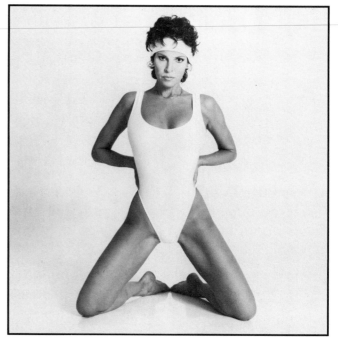

1. Place your feet together behind you, toes touching and the knees wide apart. Place your hands on your lower back.

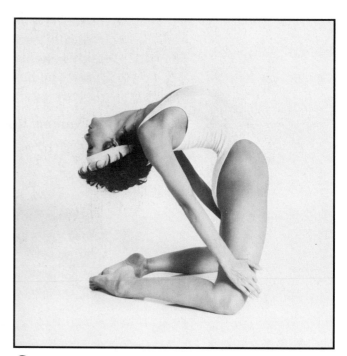

2. Inhale; drop your head all the way and arch your back. Then, bring your hands to the front of the thighs and hold on to them, pressing the pelvis and hips forward.

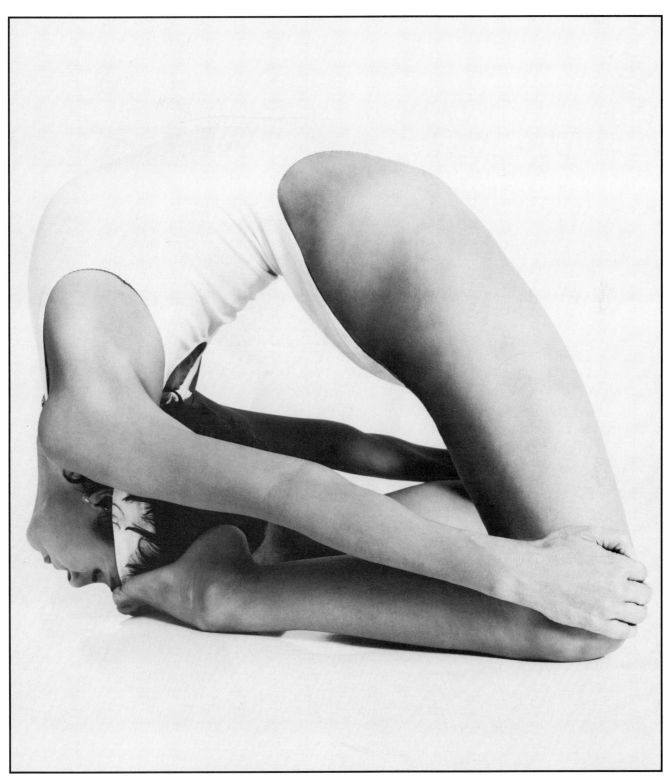

3. Once you are already arched back and holding your thighs, inch your fingers farther down to the knees, arching back all the way. Pull against your knees as you go and drop your head completely, placing it on your upturned feet. Stay for 20 seconds if you can, and come up *as slowly as possible* to allow your body to adjust.

PREPARATION

The Rabbit is a preparation for the inverted poses, so besides its many other benefits it compensates for the backward arch of the Camel Pose and is an indispensable link between that and the Shoulder Stand to come. Each step is important to make progress. Even advanced students need these preparations in order to move forward.

Benefits

- Stretches and limbers the spine, legs, and feet.
- Tones and strengthens the muscles of the neck, shoulders, back, and legs.
- Increases blood circulation to the face, the brain, and the thyroid and parathyroid glands.
- Conditions and prepares the body for the next posture, the Shoulder Stand/Plough.

A word of caution: People with high blood pressure or heart trouble should practice the Rabbit only under qualified supervision and the approval of their doctor or therapist. If you feel any discomfort, you should discontinue.

The Rabbit

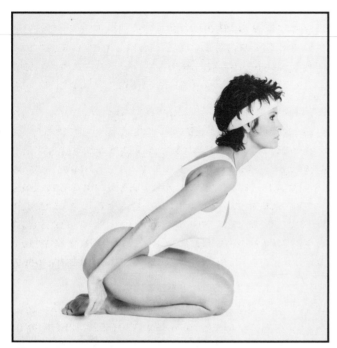

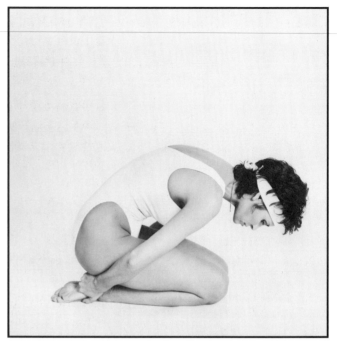

1. Sit on your heels, feet together, arms at the side. Lean forward, keeping your hips touching the heels. Reach back with your hands to the feet behind you.

2. Round your back and tip your head forward while taking hold of your heels with your hands.

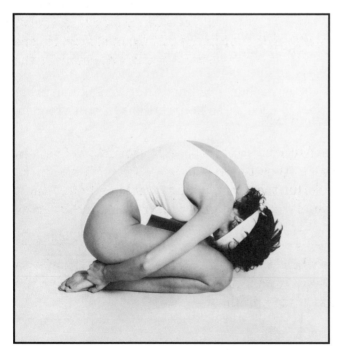

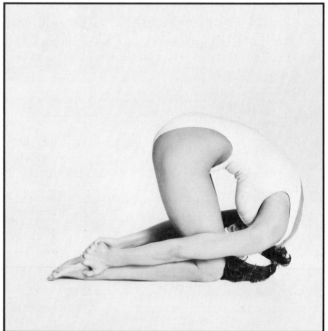

3. Your hands should grip the heels with the fingers toward the inside, thumbs on the outside. Drop your head down to touch the knees or the floor in front of them.

4. Pull hard on your heels and roll forward until the top of your head touches the floor. If your head won't touch the knees, walk your knees in toward the head when you can. Put more weight on your arms, very little on the head and neck. Hold for 20 seconds, breathe normally. Come up slowly, rest for 20 seconds. REPEAT.

Extra Help

1. The Grip. Once you get a hold on those feet, don't let go. This is the object of the whole posture. Pulling back firmly against the heels and keeping your feet flat on the floor is what holds the whole thing together. So concentrate on that above everything else.

2. Roll Forward. The roll forward of your body against your grip is what makes the spine stretch out. But don't go to extremes. If you leave a space between the head and the knees at first, that's fine—don't be discouraged. You'll work up to that when you're ready. If you've had an accident or injury to the spine, easy does it. There's no need to force yourself. Remember not to put much weight on the head and neck; take the pressure in your arms and lift the hips up. Also remember to tuck the chin in before starting the roll. It helps to curl forward correctly into the best final position.

3. Slipping. If you feel your hands slipping, come up immediately. We certainly don't want you to roll forward suddenly onto your neck. A trick my teacher taught me was to flip the corners of my towel back over my feet before even sitting down on my heels. That way, when I reached back for my feet to start the pose, the towel acted as a sort of anti-slip device.

4. Coming Up. If you've had enough before reaching the count of 20, come up and rest. Many people, myself included, feel a bit lightheaded in this pose. Build up to the full count slowly. No one expects you to do everything perfectly for the full count in the beginning. Work up to it.

Words of Encouragement

There is no need to strain in this pose. Do not attempt to push to your limit. The object is to stretch the spine out vertebra by vertebra. It's wonderful therapy for back problems and I use it myself when I'm out of whack. But do so ever so slowly and carefully.

Remember, this is a preparation for the next posture. So don't try to perform the whole play in the first act. Take it a step at a time, and you'll be able eventually to curl up into the Rabbit and come out of it feeling like a million!

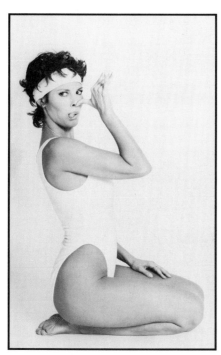

Above: *No one expects you to do everything perfectly in the beginning, so lighten up on yourself and keep your sense of humor.*

REJUVENATION

The Shoulder Stand/Plough is designed to relieve you of the symptoms of fatigue and premature aging—which, I suppose, is why many people have come to think of it as a sort of Fountain of Youth. There are actually many other postures with the facility to revitalize, invigorate, and rejuvenate you, but the Shoulder Stand combines them all in one.

It particularly focuses on the thyroid and parathyroid glands, which are positioned at the base of the neck and are stimulated by pressing your chin into the base of your throat, thereby increasing circulation to that area. It also serves to aid the function of the pineal and pituitary glands, which rest in the skull, by supplying a measured flow of blood and oxygen to the head. This is a fancy way of stating that these vital glands are treated to a rare stimulation by simply changing the flow of gravity in the body.

Benefits

Shoulder Stand (steps 1–5)

- Enhances and stimulates all vital organs of the body.
- Strengthens and limbers the upper spine.
- By reversing the blood circulation, removes fatigue and eases tension—especially relieves the heart and lungs.
- Improves menstrual irregularities and disorders.
- Helps prevent hypertension, irritability, nervousness, and insomnia.

Caution: People suffering from high blood pressure *should not* attempt this pose without checking first with their physician. They may, therefore, pass over it and do the second half, the Plough, which can help relieve this condition.

Plough (steps 6–15)

- Same basic benefits as the Shoulder Stand.
- Adds flexibility to the spine, neck, shoulders, and elbows.
- Helps relieve lumbago and arthritis of the back.
- Stimulates the internal organs by toning the stomach area.

Shoulder Stand

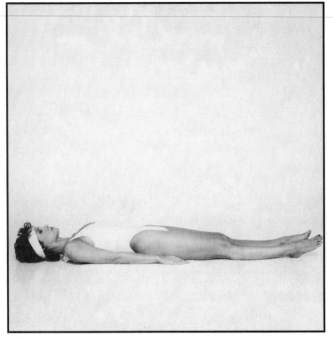

1. Take the full time to relax between the preceding pose and this one. Your body needs a chance to equalize. Then, turn your palms to the floor.

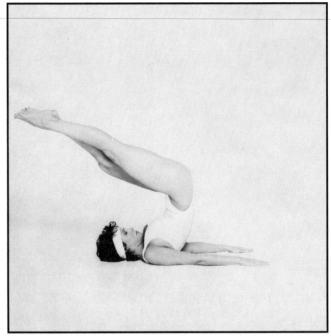

2. Pressing against the floor with your hands, take a deep breath and swing your legs up over your head—one leg, then the other. If you need to bend your legs going up, that's okay.

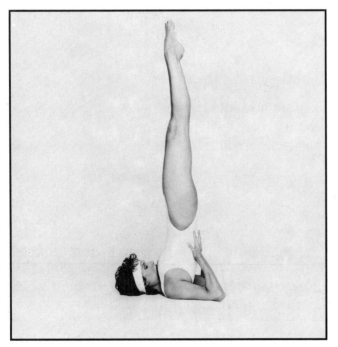

3. As you swing up, bring your hands in to support your back. Press your elbows against the floor and lift your body and legs up as far as is comfortable. Hold for 10 seconds. Center your chin and neck.

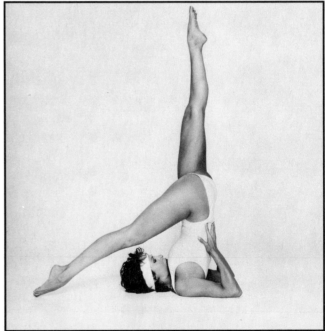

4. Keeping your back supported, lower your right leg and touch the floor behind you. Do not, however, sacrifice a straight back to do so. It's better not to touch than round your spine. Hold for 10 seconds.

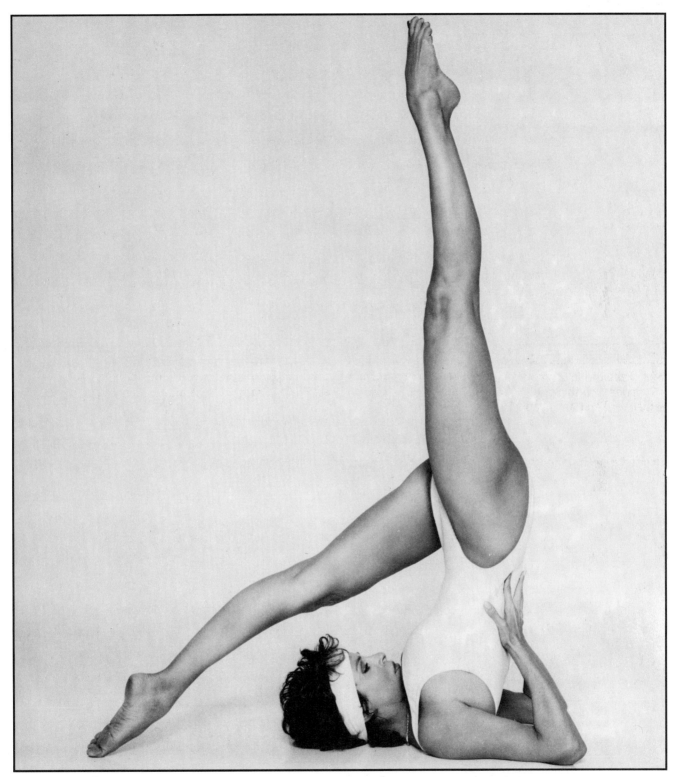

5. After bringing your right leg back up, lower your left leg to the floor. Hold for 10 counts. Then, bring the leg back up to join the other. Keep stretching your body up from your shoulders to the toes. If you feel discomfort in the shoulders and neck, roll slowly out of the pose at once.

Plough

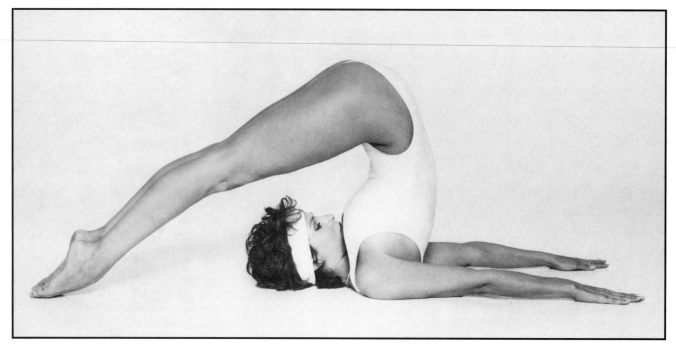

6. Lower both legs together over your head and touch your feet to the floor behind you. Hold for 10 counts. You have the option of leaving your hands on your back for support or stretching your arms behind you, as seen above. Make yourself secure and comfortable in this inverted posture.

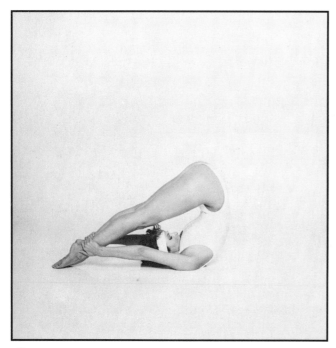

8. To come out, or roll out, take hold of your feet, straighten your legs and begin to curl your back down onto the floor, vertebra by vertebra.

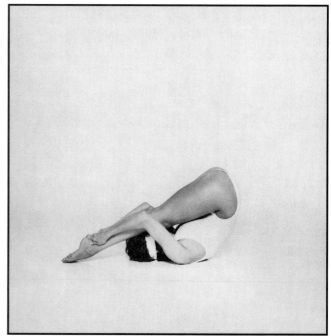

9. As you are executing your reverse curl, pull your legs to your face and body for an extra stretch. Make sure your chin is centered throughout this pose.

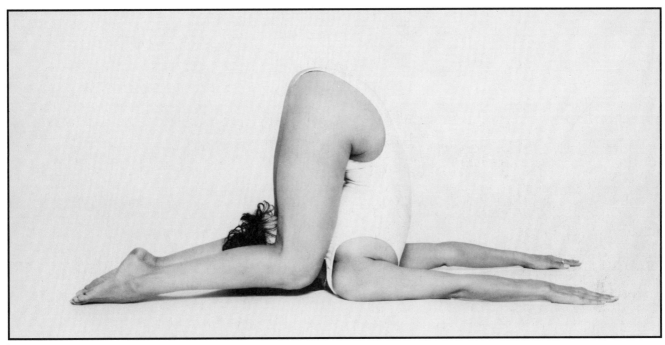

7. Now, open your knees and slowly lower them to the floor beside your head. Hold 10 counts. If you have difficulty or experience discomfort at any point in this sequence, don't hesitate to roll out of the pose.

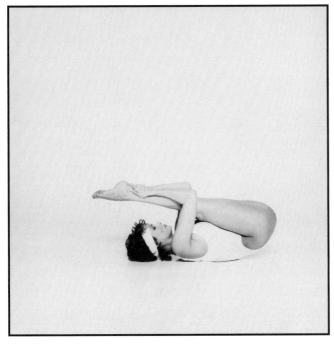

10. When your back is on the floor again, you can allow your legs to pull away from your body and release the pull of the arms.

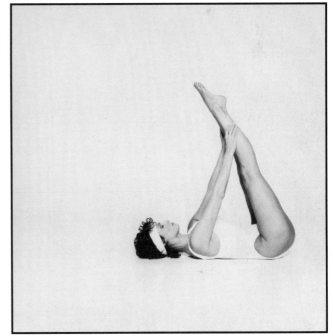

11. Continue to lower your legs until your hips are all the way down on the floor. Make this a *very slow process*. Remember you are coming out of an inverted pose. Your body must readjust.

Plough

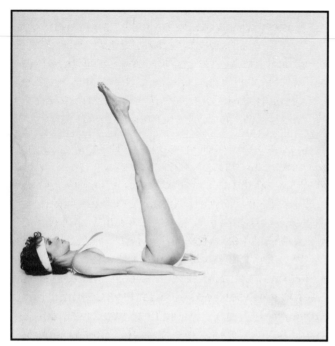

12. Place your arms at your sides, pressing against the floor with your hands, and proceed to lower your legs. It's also acceptable to place your hands under the buttocks while lowering the legs.

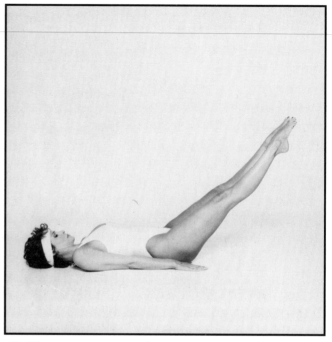

13. At this point, your abdominals come more into play, so use your stomach muscles.

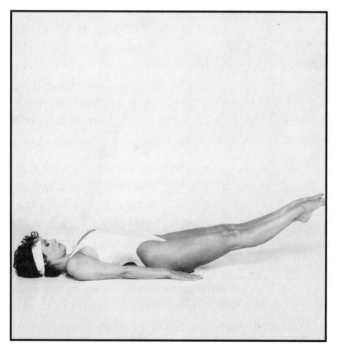

14. When your legs get within 6 to 12 inches of the floor, hold them there for 10 counts. Use the strength of your arms as well as the abdominals. Don't strain your back.

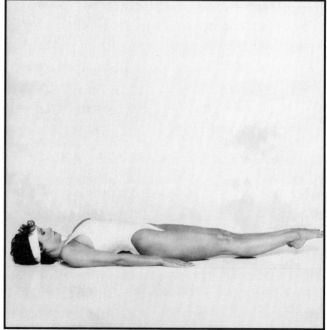

15. Finally, let your feet touch the floor. Relax for *30 seconds.* Advanced students may substitute this pose for the second set of the Rabbit. *Do not repeat!*

Extra Help

1. Caution. Small wonder that with so much to gain from this posture, it takes regular practice and caution to perform it correctly. Therefore, if at any point during the course of this cycle you feel tension or discomfort in the neck and shoulders, back off a bit. Far better to be comfortable in these inverted positions and add steps gradually than to go too far and cause injury.

2. Going Up. For most people there's something spooky about being upside down, because your body needs to adjust to the change in gravity. So it is very important to *relax* into the pose when you first feel the weight of your body resting on the shoulders and neck. I've suffered many injuries to this area, so I know how it can feel. If it's too much, roll out (see paragraph 10 below); rest, and then try again. I did, and eventually I could go up without the discomfort. However, *don't lift* past the first stage, when your legs are at a 45-degree angle, until you feel good in that position and have established slow, steady breathing. Then, and only then, should you proceed to lift your back, hips, and legs high into the vertical position. Once again, *relax* in the final pose, *eyes wide open and breathing gently and easily. Never, never jerk or flop into or out of this pose.*

3. High Blood Pressure. For those of you who have a tendency to high blood pressure, put aside the Shoulder Stand and concentrate first on the Plough. Proficiency in the Plough can help this condition. Also, by doing the Plough first, followed by the Shoulder Stand, you may avoid the feeling of blood rushing to the head; the Plough can be used as a preparation for the more advanced Shoulder Stand. However, I want to stress again that high blood pressure patients not attempt the Shoulder Stand without a doctor's advice and a qualified instructor present.

4. Legs. Once you're all the way up, there is a tendency for the legs to swing out of the perpendicular line. To prevent this, tighten the muscles at the back of the thighs and buttocks and stretch the length of your body upward, letting the legs sway back a little.

5. Falling. In the beginning, some people get the feeling that they'll fall over; I've had it myself, but I never did. Try to reassure yourself that this is a normal sensation. But if you can't shake it, and it's making you tense, do the Shoulder Stand in a corner of the room where your feet can touch the wall for added security. If you're having great difficulty, it would be preferable to have a qualified instructor present.

Shoulder Stand/Plough

6. Elbows. From the start, the elbows should not be placed wider than the shoulders. Then, once you're all the way up in the vertical position, try to ease them closer together while stretching your shoulders away from the neck. If the elbows are too wide, the torso cannot be held in the straight-up position, and the pose will appear imperfect from the profile. It should be at right angles to the floor.

7. Chin Lock. Pressing your chin into the base of your throat causes a choking sensation. Don't panic. This is absolutely normal. Remind yourself of all the good it is doing the thyroid glands; relax and allow your breathing to adapt. This chin lock encourages deep abdominal breathing. Be sure to press the chin to the chest and not the other way around. Do not bring the chest up to the chin— or you will miss the full benefit of the pose. Check to see that the back of your neck is completely flat on the floor and relax that area as much as possible. It is also *very important to make sure that your neck is straight.* In the beginning, it has a tendency to move sideways to counteract the unaccustomed pressure. Be sure that your chin is resting on the center of your upper chest. If you relax and concentrate, you will avoid unnecessary pain and injury.

8. Eyes Open. Throughout this inverted position, keep your eyes open and your mind in the present. Do not allow yourself to drift off. This is as controlled and precise as any posture in the series.

9. Limitations. *Under no circumstances exceed your limitations.* If you cannot get all the way up, don't force yourself. Easy does it. If you can get all the way up to the vertical position, but cannot stay very long, come down and rest. Do not be discouraged, but do try again. Use the allotted time in this pose to good advantage. You'll get it before too long.

10. Roll-out. If at any time you suffer discomfort and want to come out of the pose, always use the roll-out. It is important to come out of the pose as slowly as you went in. First, lower your legs to a 45-degree angle over your head, place your palms flat on the floor beside you, and de-contract your spine, vertebra by vertebra. Breathe normally throughout, until your entire spine is resting on the floor and your legs are perpendicular to it. Then exhale and slowly lower your straight legs down to the floor.

11. The Plough. When performing this pose, concentrate on keeping your spine stretched up while your knees remain straight. Your feet may not reach the floor at first, but as your spine becomes more flexible, the weight of your legs alone will gradually bring them down.

12. Rest Period. More advanced students may go right into the Plough from the Shoulder Stand. However, if you feel too much strain you may relax in between these two movements. Use the roll-out, of course, to come down.

Words of Encouragement

Wouldn't you know that a pose with so much gold would require a lot of digging. Most people are familiar with the Shoulder Stand but it is deceptively difficult to do correctly. Indeed, you may be among those for whom the Shoulder Stand is *not* indicated. This is nothing against you. It is, in fact, rather common, and is why the famous, and more advanced, Head Stand is not offered in this program.

In the final analysis, the Shoulder Stand is nice to have, but you don't *need* it. You can achieve the same benefits through the combination of the other postures. In my experience, it took over five years to get it right and I'm a pretty strict taskmaster. So just move on to the Plough and rest assured that respecting your body's limitations is by far the better part of valor.

Who knows? At another time, like me, you may come back to it and find you can do it without difficulty. On the other hand, if *you can* do it, you *should*. It comes in very handy in this hectic world as a pick-me-upper.

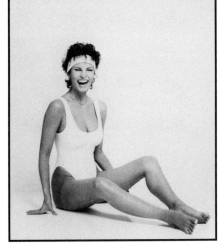

Above: *I have good reason to be laughing here. It took me a long time to work up to the Shoulder Stand. Now when I roll out of it I feel like a million.*

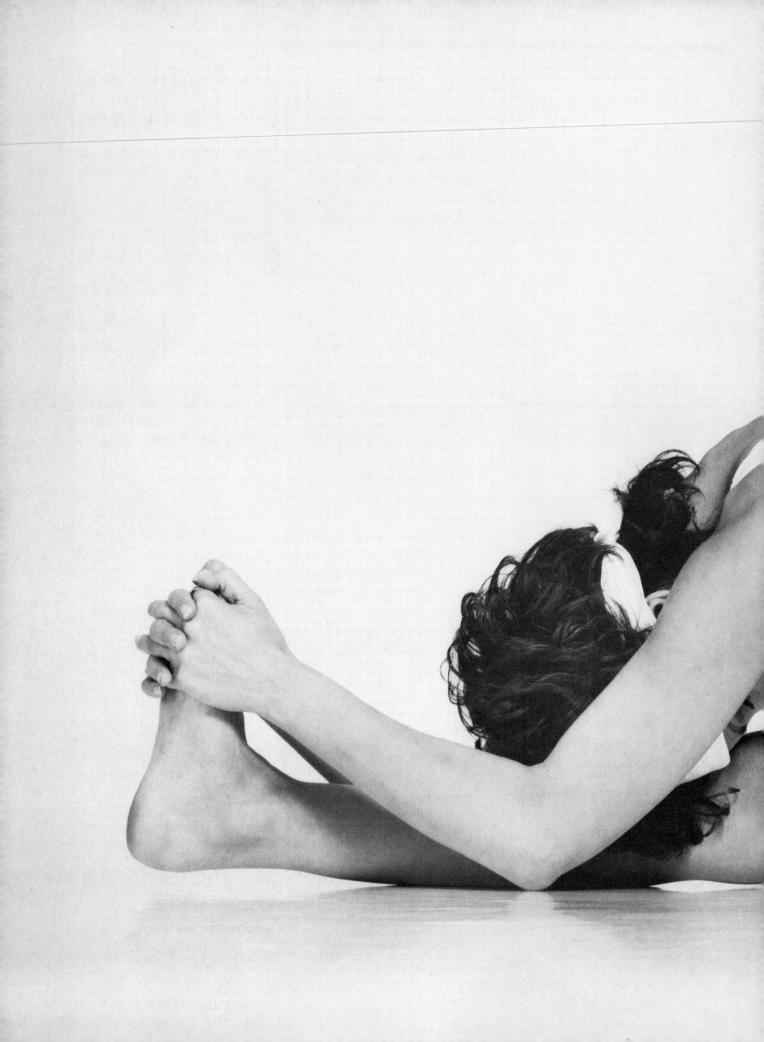

FLEXIBILITY

The Stretching Cycle

You can walk away feeling lithe, limber, and lighter on your feet than you have since you were a small kid.

At this stage of the game, we're rounding the last bend in the road. The class is almost over. So you'll probably be relieved and quite relaxed. Since relaxation is important to these final stretches—use it. It will serve you well. The Stretching Cycle ahead is a final chance to reaffirm the flexibility you have gained all through the routine. And now too comes the payoff for the series of smart swing-ups you've been doing at the end of all the kneeling postures. Prepare for the final stretches so you can walk away feeling lithe, limber, and lighter on your feet than you have since you were a small kid.

Benefits

Head to Knee (steps 1–4)

- Strengthens and tones the abdominal organs, including the spleen, kidneys, colon, and adrenal glands.
- Stretches and works the back and the legs, limbers the hip, knee, and ankle joints, and relaxes the hamstrings.
- Improves and helps digestion.

Full Stretch (steps 5–9)

- Fully stretches the body, from the neck to the feet, especially the lower spine area and the muscles of the shoulders, upper arms, back, and legs.
- Tones the hip joints and the nerves and ligaments of the legs, and makes them more flexible.
- Improves and slims the waistline and tightens the abdomen.
- Massages and invigorates the abdominal organs, particularly the kidneys, spleen, stomach, and liver.
- Helps relieve and cure digestive disorders.

Spread Eagle (steps 10–13)

- Stretches and increases the elasticity of the spine, and the back and leg muscles, ligaments, and tendons.
- Conditions and works the inner thighs and calves.
- Helps relieve and prevent hernia and sciatic pains.
- Controls and improves menstrual irregularities or disorders.

Head to Knee

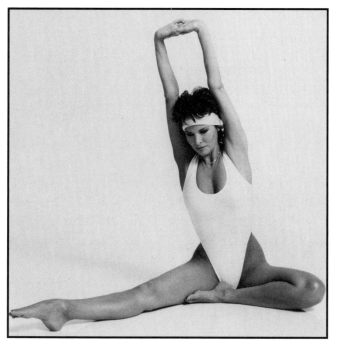

1. Sit with your hips on the floor and extend your right leg. Bend the left one and place the bottom of the foot in the corner of the right upper thigh. Stretch your arms up over your head, interlace your fingers, and turn them inside out. Now, stretch out over the extended leg.

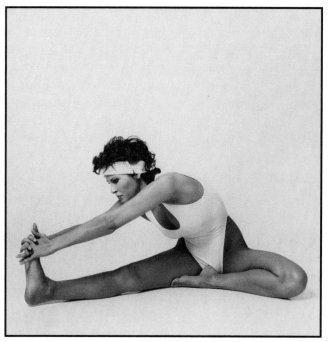

2. Now, reach forward and place the stirrup of your hands over the ball of your flexed foot.

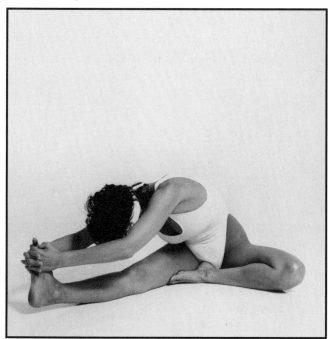

3. Pull against your foot, lifting the heel off the floor if you can, and drop your chin toward your chest.

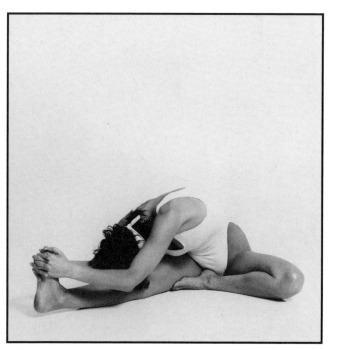

4. Still pulling back on your foot, so you feel the stretch, drop your head to the knee and your elbows to the floor, beside the leg. Stay for 10 counts. Come up slowly and then do the other side.

Full Stretch

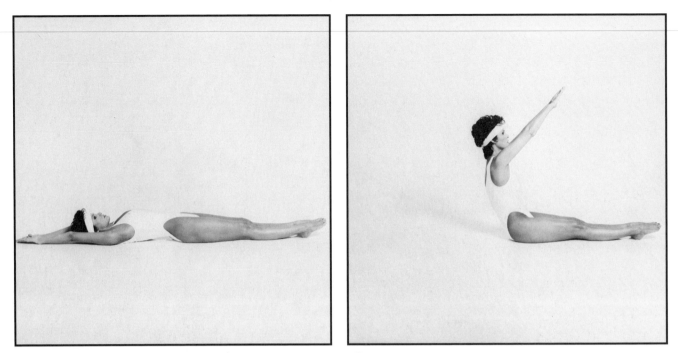

5. Without delay, lie back on the floor and get ready for a Swing-Up, hands together over the head and toes pointed.

6. Inhale and come up swiftly and immediately by swinging the arms forward.

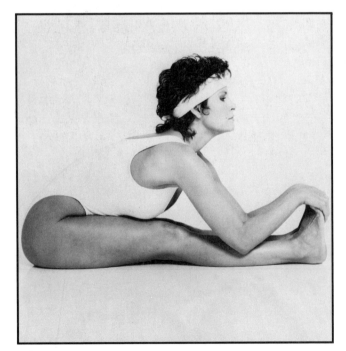

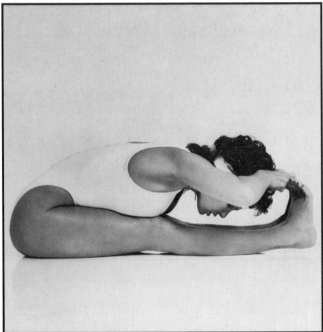

7. Grab hold of the toes as you have done before in each Swing-Up, between postures. Scoot your hips out behind you—left-right, left-right—and stretch forward even more.

8. Wrap the first 2 fingers of each hand around the big toes (see Extra Help). Now, on an exhale, pull the heels right up off the floor while pulling your toes toward the top of your head.

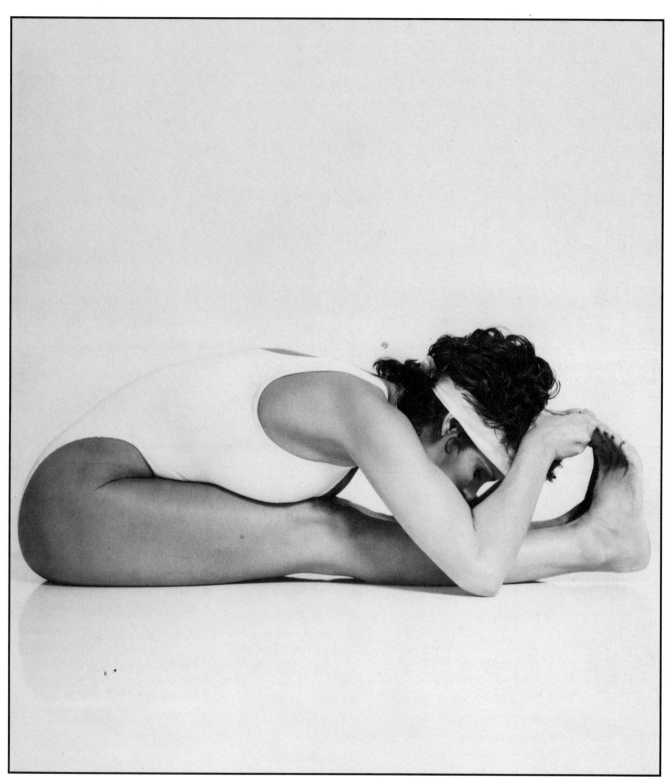

9. Lower your elbows to the floor. Concentrate on the exhalation, keep pulling gently but firmly, and feel your legs and spine release gradually. Hold for 20 slow counts. Breathe and relax into it. Rest, swing up, and REPEAT the Head to Knee and Full Stretch (steps 1–9) before proceeding to step 10.

Spread Eagle

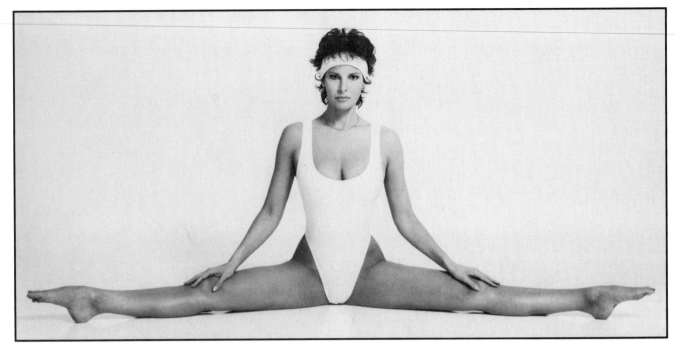

10. Spread your legs as wide to the side as possible, sitting on both hips evenly. This is the final stretching pose of the cycle.

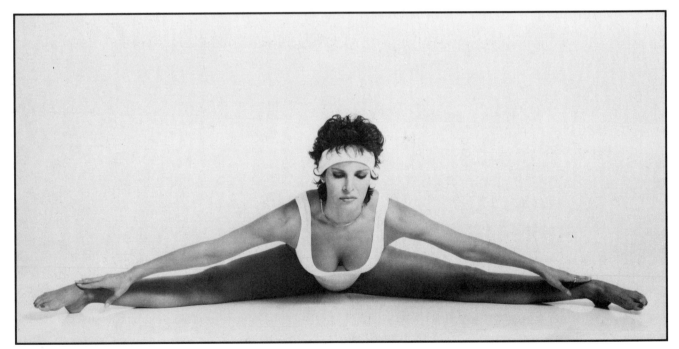

12. Continue to lower yourself toward the floor, your hands moving farther along the legs. If you don't yet have the flexibility to do this, place your hands on the floor in front of you and walk yourself down.

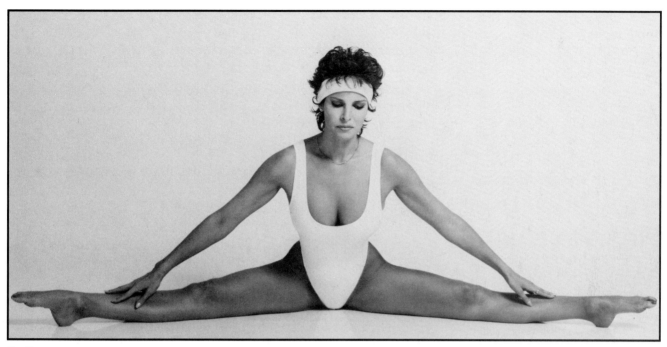

11. Placing your hands on the legs, bend your body forward in a straight line from the hips, allowing your legs to rotate slightly inward as you go.

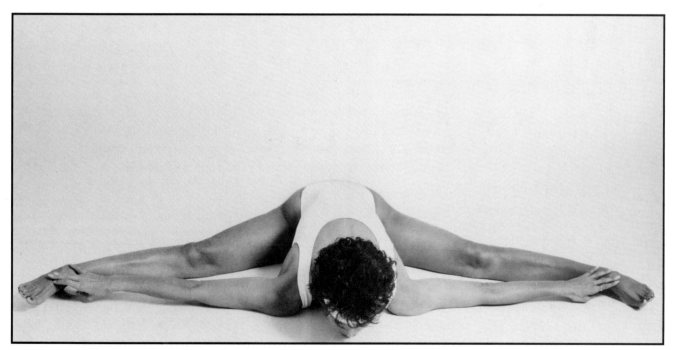

13. When you finally get down this far, your legs have become flexible enough to put your chin on the floor. But that doesn't happen in one day! Don't rush it. If need be, support yourself on your elbows and concentrate on exhalation. Hold your best position faithfully and relax. Inevitably, flexibility will come. *Do not repeat this pose.*

The Stretching Cycle

Extra Help

1. Final Stretch. You will be sufficiently warmed up by this time to do these last postures without much difficulty. Not that any beginner is expected to just lie down on top of their legs like in the photos. But it's important to give this cycle all the attention it deserves to finish things off nicely and take advantage of all your hard work so far.

2. Each Day. You'll find that you become more flexible quickly, if you practice regularly; and you'll look upon this stretching cycle as just another ounce of good measure to keep you that way.

Head to Knee

1. Can't Reach. If you can't reach your feet either in the single-leg stretch or the full forward one, bend the knees and take hold of your feet. Then try to straighten them. If you have difficulty doing that, concentrate on pushing forward with the heel while pulling back against the toes, just as you did in the Standing Head to Knee posture (Number 5) at the beginning. Now you have a chance to practice this movement without the need to balance.

2. Lopsided. If you're worried about being lopsided, don't panic. Everyone is like that. It's just more noticeable in some poses than others.

3. Patience. Don't compare yourself with the photos and start to judge yourself. They are the results of all the efforts I'm advising you to do. Your progress will be measured in inches that add up to a lot in the end.

4. Tips. I used to do this stretch after getting out of a hot tub, so I could make faster headway. It works, but not in a single day. The only thing that insures results is knowing that you can do it and giving it your very best shot as often as possible.

5. Swing-Up. *Do* swing out over your legs briskly and grab hold of your toes. Again, if you can't reach all the way, hold what you can. But don't give up.

Full Stretch

1. Relax. Do relax and exhale forward in this forward stretch, regardless of any doubts or misgivings about ever reaching your feet, much less touching them to your head. Be as skeptical as you want, but keep at it. Scoot your hips back, push those heels forward and pull against your toes. Press your head to the knees and try to get them to straighten against the floor, and remember that when you have problems and work through them, you are making the most progress.

Spread Eagle

A good stretch is like a yawn—if you don't complete it you feel unsatisfied.

1. **Legs Wide.** Your legs are slightly rotated in this forward stretch and are stretched by the weight of your body. Get them as far apart as possible—but take it easy. Slow but sure is the best policy.

2. **Walking Down.** Under no circumstance should you flop down, even if you are very limber. Everything in yoga is very graceful and controlled.

3. **Chin and Chest.** Since you have to stay in the position for 20 seconds, find the maximum point you can support comfortably for that time. While you're there, concentrate on exhalation and you will release farther from the lower back and inner thigh naturally. So take your time. Let your body do the work. You have to be at the maximum point, though—no cheating.

4. **Toehold.** Don't attempt this until you are well down and can hold the position with chin and chest on the floor for 20 counts. Then progress further, taking hold of the toes and pulling them to the floor.

5. **Coming Up.** Come up slowly, little by little—as you went down. There's no reason even for an expert to risk injury by sloppy procedure.

Words of Encouragement

I've heard it said that a good stretch is like a yawn—if you don't complete it you feel unsatisfied. Your body wants to stretch and release; so let it do so without aggravation. Be a spectator to your body's reactions; you'll be delighted to discover the innate intelligence it has, in this and all the postures. Direct it but don't force it. It teaches you how to treat yourself in real life. Friendly persuasion is worth a thousand orders at gunpoint.

Once you're finally down and stretched, ah . . . what a feeling, it's absolute bliss. That's why you'll get there. Your body is no fool, it senses something good lies ahead.

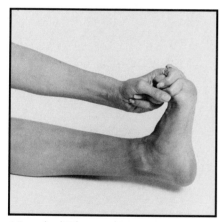

Above: *This is the toehold described in step 8 of the Full Stretch pose. Wrap the first two fingers of each hand around your big toes and close your thumb over them.*

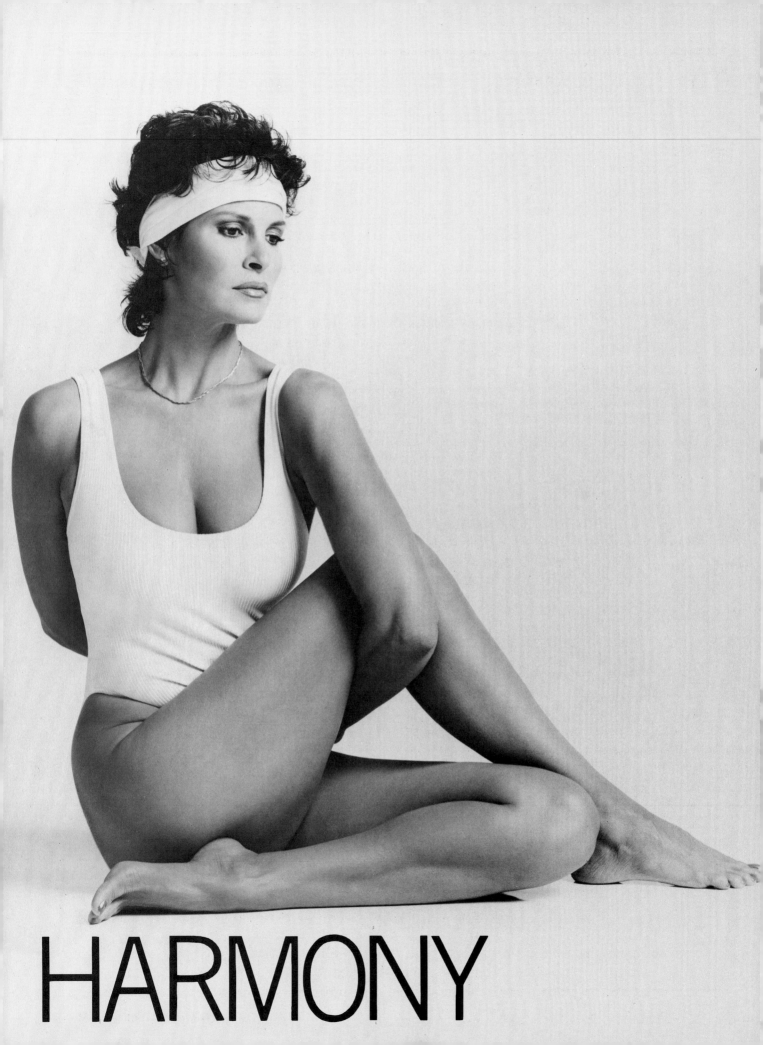

HARMONY

The Spinal Twist

This is the final twist. After stretching your body, both forward and back, the moment has now arrived to rotate the spine and refresh and realign yourself before finishing the series. It has a sort of winding-down effect.

At this point, you'll notice that you're not at all weary from your previous efforts. The Spinal Twist is part of this revitalizing process, so by the time you're done, you'll be lively and alert.

Benefits

- Fully develops the elasticity of the spine in a twisting motion.
- Tightens and firms the muscles of the neck, abdomen, buttocks, and thighs and breaks down superfluous fat.
- Limbers the hip and shoulder joints.
- Tones the spinal nerves and stimulates the functions of the internal organs such as the spleen, liver, kidneys, and intestines.
- Improves blood circulation and digestion.

The Spinal Twist

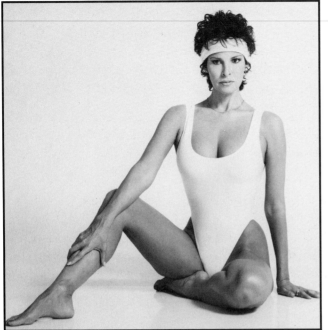

1. Sit with your weight evenly distributed on both hips. Your right foot is on the floor, with your hand resting lightly on the lower leg. Bend your left leg inward.

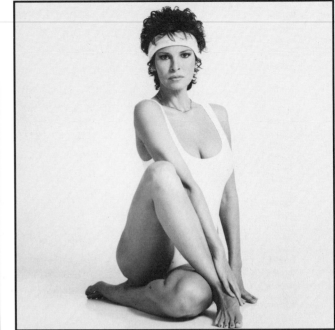

2. Now place your right leg over the left one without raising the hip off the floor, and position the foot at the knee.

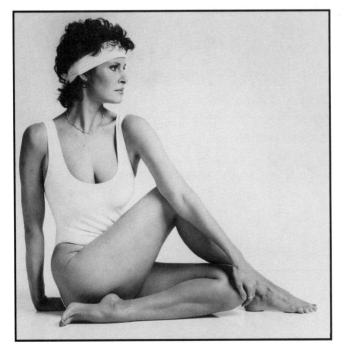

3. Switch the position of your arms. The left arm should be placed on the outside of the raised leg, with the hand fitting neatly over the kneecap of the leg underneath. The right hand rests on the floor behind the hip.

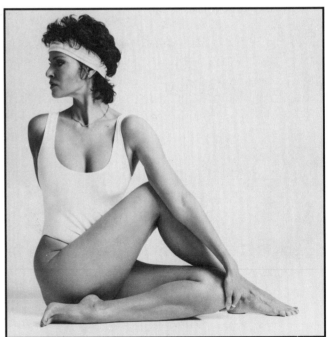

4. Twist your head and body slowly around, as far as possible. Keep your shoulders even and both hips touching the floor. Hold for 20 seconds. *Do not repeat.*

Extra Help

1. What Goes Where. It seems more complicated than it is, but once you get it, your body will remember easily and fall into it almost automatically. The first few times you do this pose, take your time to get the confusion ironed out. It's right leg over left knee, reach around it with the left arm, take hold of the knee, and look backward over your other shoulder.

2. Important Details. Check to see that *both hips sit evenly on the floor*—and press downward with the lower knee; don't let it pull up.

3. Twist. Lift your torso up and don't slouch into the pose. Then, twist around just as though your waist was a wet dishcloth and look behind yourself with your eyes. Don't try any fancy grips until you have the basics down. Nonetheless, you'll still be getting the benefits of the postures at every level of development. It's your body that counts, not the performance.

Words of Encouragement

The Spinal Twist is a classic pose that brings to mind beauty and harmony. It has a very refreshing effect so you'll enjoy giving it your full concentration. Twist away your cares and woes . . . there's only two more steps to go.

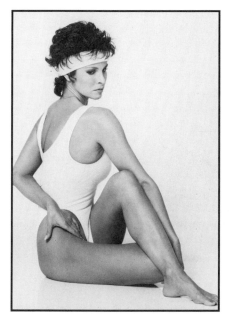

Above: *This illustrates an alternative grip for the back arm, with the hand holding on to the hip bone. Or you may just let your hand rest, palm up, on your waistline.*

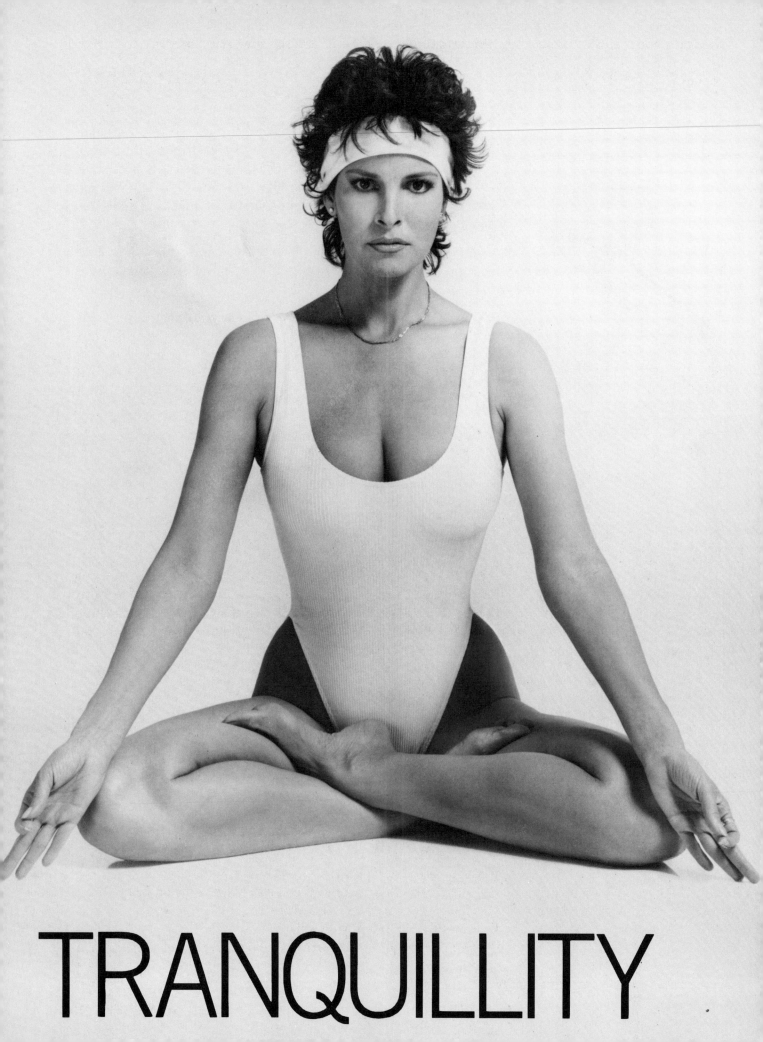

TRANQUILLITY

This is the last posture, except for the Blowing Pose. The Lotus is famous as a meditative pose, but it is also the right finishing touch for those of you who enjoy sitting quietly and evenly balanced in a relaxed state.

Aren't you relieved? All your problems and worries are behind you now. You have tackled all your demons, your doubts, and your fears. You've had an inner dialogue and looked yourself in the eye. You've made new discoveries, charted a new course. You're fully equipped and better acquainted with yourself. And you're ready to melt into the floor with a sense of relief. That's exactly what you're going to do in a few moments. Hold on, you're almost there.

Benefits

- Improves the flexibility of the hip, knee, and ankle joints.
- Stretches the thigh muscles and the sciatic nerve.
- Increases circulation to the spine, abdomen, and brain.
- Tones the entire nervous system.
- Makes deep breathing easier.
- Helps relieve and cure arthritis, rheumatism, and sciatica pains.

The Lotus

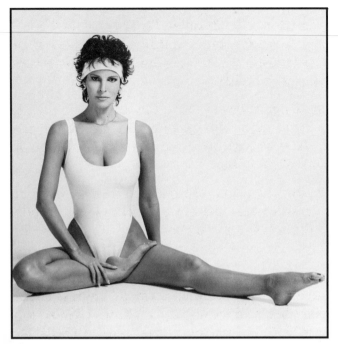

1. Sit evenly on your hips, with your back completely straight. Bend one knee in, and place the foot on the opposite thigh. Then press your bent knee down as much as possible.

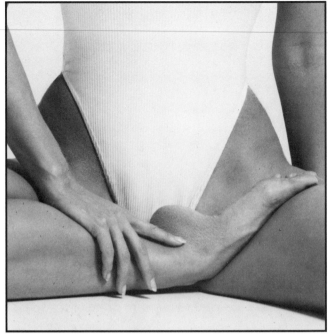

2. This closeup of Step 1 shows the exact placement of the foot on the thigh.

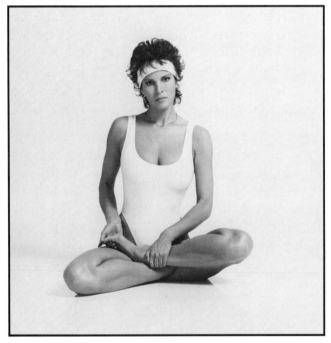

3. Now, pick up the second foot and place it on top of the opposite thigh, as high as it will go. Sit with your back erect.

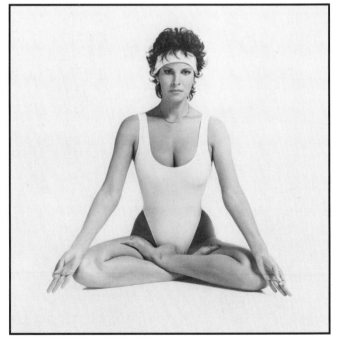

4. Both knees should touch the floor, although one knee often remains slightly up until you become more limber. Now place your hands, palms up, on the knees and touch your thumbs to the forefingers. Remain in the pose for 20 seconds. *Do not repeat.*

Extra Help

I didn't get into the full Lotus until three years ago myself—so take heart!

1. Half Lotus. If you are not yet flexible enough to do the classic Lotus, try the Half Lotus. From step 1, bring the second foot in and slip it *under* the opposite thigh. This is easier for beginners until the legs become more limber.

2. Homework One. To gain flexibility in the legs for the Lotus, you can practice at home. Sit in the position shown in step 1 and press your knee to the floor with your hand, holding it there for 20 seconds. Then do the other leg.

3. Homework Two. Sit down and, bringing the soles of your feet together—heels near the crotch—take hold of the feet and bounce your knees up and down. Try this in your spare time—it speeds your progress.

4. Knees. If stiff knees prevent you from even coming close to the Half Lotus, don't give up. Keep working away at the rest of the routine, do your homework, and eventually you'll see yourself improve. I didn't get into the full Lotus until three years ago myself—so take heart!

Words of Encouragement

Congratulations in advance for the time in your practice when everything comes into sync and you can perform the postures almost effortlessly. You can look forward to finding yourself carried along by a momentum you created with care and patience, but which now requires nothing more of you. It's terrific! Like learning to drive or ride a bicycle: once you've got it, it's yours—and you never lose it. I have confidence that you'll get it . . . see you there.

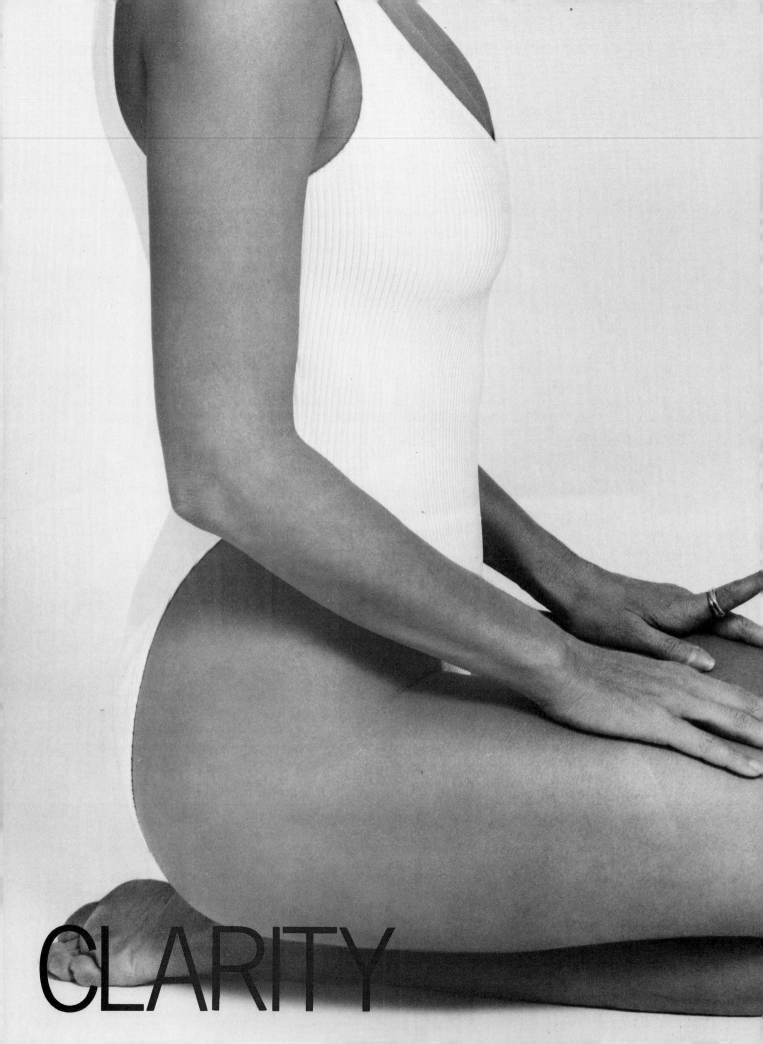

CLARITY

Blowing Pose   Number 28

In some circles, this last breathing exercise is called the *cleansing breath,* because it clears the mind and gets it out of the fog, "shining" it up to a high sheen. It revitalizes you and gets you back out into the fray, rarin' to go. You'll be newly concentrated and your sense of priorities will improve, so that you make better use of your time. It sends you out into the world "shining."

Benefits

- Cleanses and revitalizes the body.
- Rids the lower lungs of spent air and carbon dioxide, and clears the sinuses.
- Improves blood circulation.
- Activates and stimulates abdominal muscles and organs.
- Clears the mind and improves concentration.

Blowing Pose

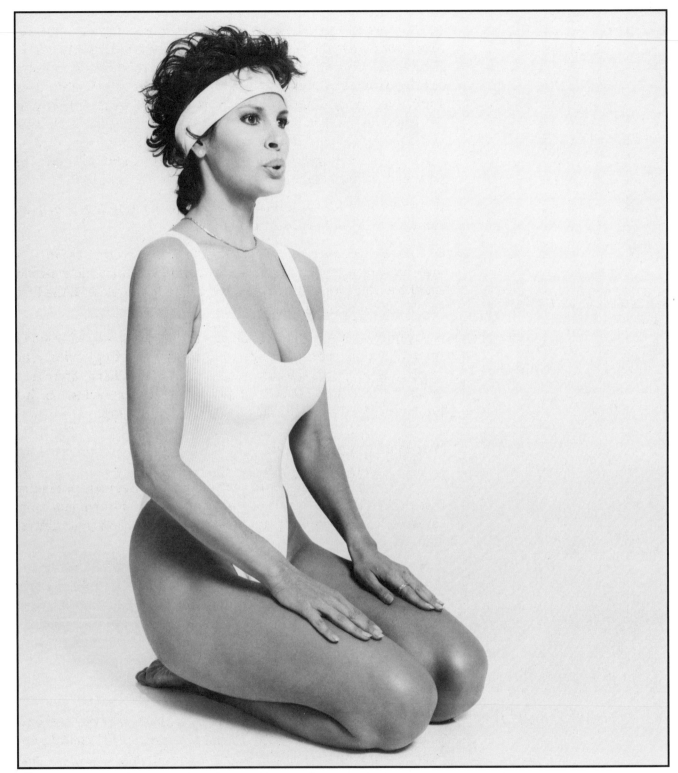

1. Sit on your heels and allow your stomach to relax *out*. Then, synchronize blowing *out* sharply while you pull *in* with your stomach muscles. Continue to *contract your abdominals*, in time with your blowing. Meanwhile, count sets of 10 on your fingers, keeping the tempo fairly brisk, until you reach 60. Rest and then REPEAT a second set of 60.

Extra Help

1. **Synchronizing.** The key to this breathing pose is to synchronize blowing *out* sharply with contracting the stomach muscles *in*. It takes a couple of rounds to get used to, but most people are able to fall into the rhythm. Start with your stomach relaxed *out;* place your hand on it so you can feel the muscles working as they pull in. Then, blow out and pull in at the same time. After each blow the stomach automatically comes back *out* again. So keep on blowing and contracting, setting up a steady even count. Concentrate on the exhaling because the inhaling takes care of itself.

2. **Isolation.** This is an isolation exercise. *Nothing* moves but the stomach. Hold yourself steady and work it.

3. **Tired.** If you should become lightheaded or dizzy before the first set is over, stop and relax. Then, start again and do a second set of the same amount that you were able to complete in the first set. Work up to more gradually.

4. **Counting.** My teacher taught me an ingenious way of keeping track of the breaths as you blow. Just tap your thigh with your finger, starting with the little finger of your right hand, and count to ten; for the next set of 10, tap the next finger; and so on. It's fun and helps you concentrate on what you're doing.

Words of Encouragement

So now you have come to the end of the road; your prizes are rest and relaxation. Lie down on your back and abandon your cares, leaving them far behind. Nothing can disturb you, time is yours.

The Last Word

I don't know about you, but I'm exhausted, relieved, and satisfied I've done my best. I hope that these postures help to enhance your life as they have mine. They are here for the asking, so take them and use them for all they are worth. God bless you.

Special Payoffs

By this time you know that there are a cornucopia of benefits that can be gained as a result of this daily routine. But what you don't know about yet are the special payoffs that are in store for you as well.

Physical Benefits

1. The Gentle Body Builder

In my experience, this method is the only physical activity that can actually change your body construction and rearrange your anatomy from what you start out with. As my yoga teacher, Bikram, used to say, it remolds your shape in much the same way a blacksmith makes horseshoes—heating up the iron before bending it into the desired shape.

First you heat the body by scientific stretching, thus making it pliable. Then you remold it by holding the positions steady, aligning every muscle, ligament, and tendon in your framework so that all of your proportions are in balance. With this technique even your bone structure can be changed. We tend to think of bones as being brittle—but they're not cement. In fact, one woman I know actually realigned and straightened her bowlegs! Incredible? Yes, but I've seen it happen often enough, with people of all shapes and sizes, that I've come to accept it as almost commonplace.

As you progress, your own proportions will dictate the changes that are necessary to bring about a better and more beautiful body within your physical framework. If your bone structure is faulty, these postures will help to correct that as well.

2. A Natural Face-lift

What would you say if I told you that this method and the proper diet—which is a natural offshoot of it—are the equivalent of a natural face-lift? Would you sit up and take notice? Ah ha. Gotcha!

It's a popular misconception that certain signs of aging, such as puffy eyes and a sagging chin line, are irreversible. This is just not true. They are merely signs of neglect. Need I remind you that *your head is attached to your body*? So if you're using this method, the whole thing improves; it doesn't stop at the neck. Isn't that good news?

It's a popular misconception that certain signs of aging, such as puffy eyes and a sagging chin line, are irreversible. This is just not true. They are merely signs of neglect.

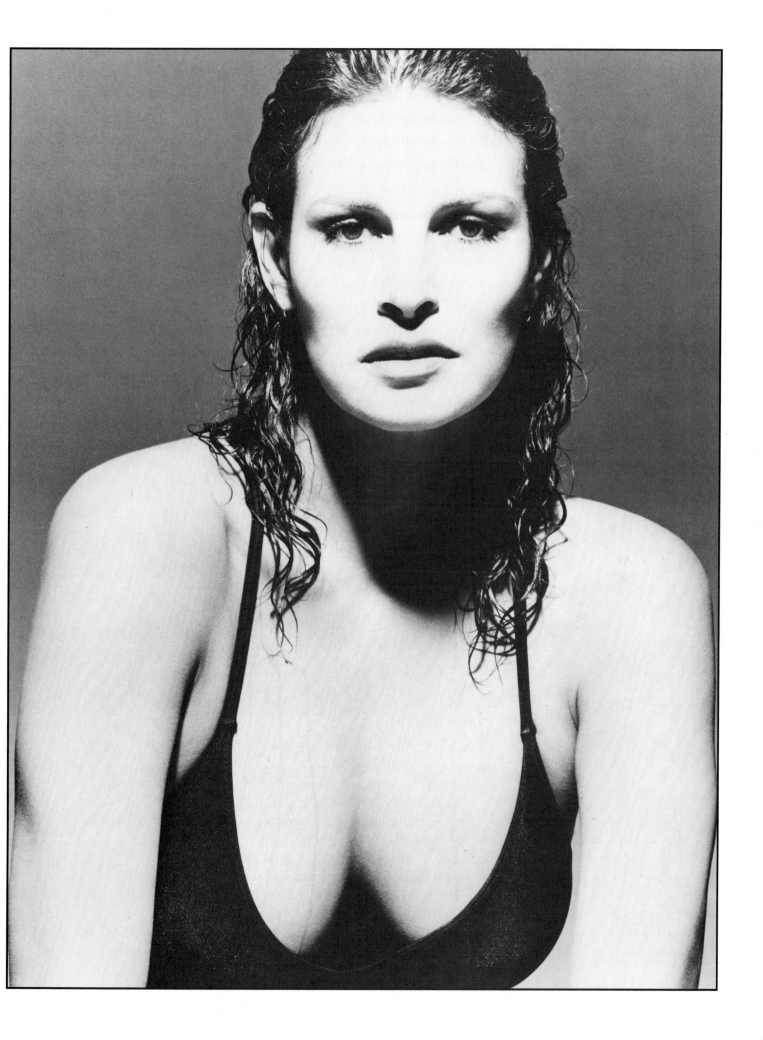

You would be amazed at the amount of cosmetic surgery that is absolutely unnecessary, simply because so much can be accomplished with diet and exercise.

Below: *Stress is the good guy—distress is the culprit! Here a lady in distress is about to become a basket case* (The Three Musketeers).

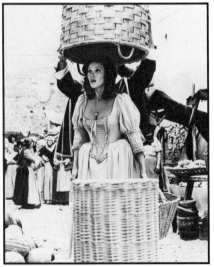

Almost immediately, you will begin to notice that your face has more color and that, as your flesh settles into its natural facial contours, the fine lines around your eyes and mouth become less noticeable. When you lose weight your skin will not look slack because these postures are stimulating glands and hormones most other programs miss. This routine also teaches you to control the facial muscles so that tension and effort are not expressed through wrinkled brows and grimaces.

Granted, it's harder pedaling uphill than it is taking the downhill slide into a surgeon's office. But you would be amazed at the amount of cosmetic surgery that is absolutely unnecessary, simply because so much can be accomplished with diet and exercise alone!

It never ceases to astonish me that some of the same women who find a regular exercise routine insupportable wouldn't bat an eyelash at submitting to, among other things, the "black and blue" school of massage therapy, having staples stuck in their ears, body wraps, and overdoses of diuretics, not to mention regular visits to the plastic surgeon.

The risk of disfigurement and the countless humiliations involved in *unneeded* cosmetic surgery should be enough to scare most people away. But the idea of putting ourselves into the hands of an "expert" is virtually irresistible. So do yourself a favor, and think twice about it.

Mental Benefits

1. Active Relaxation

For the past few years, we've heard of nothing if we haven't heard of *stress*. It has occurred to me, however, that without stress of some kind we'd all be incapable of standing up straight—we'd become limp in mind and body. We need stress, in fact, to function—it's fundamental to the balance of things.

What the commotion is all about, then, is *dis*tress. To break it down further: stress is the good guy, distress is the culprit. To alleviate distress we need only subtract the "dis"—or active negativity—keep that stress which sustains our drive, and *voilà*! . . . you are free of distress.

The catch is that, sometimes, even after the cause of distress is removed, the imprint of the experience remains in the body, almost like scar tissue. And unless these residual effects are taken care of properly, they can cause chronic problems, such as "executive necks," migraines, muscle spasms, backaches, and the like.

Enter active relaxation, a by-product of this daily routine. It first relieves distress and second establishes a state of well-being

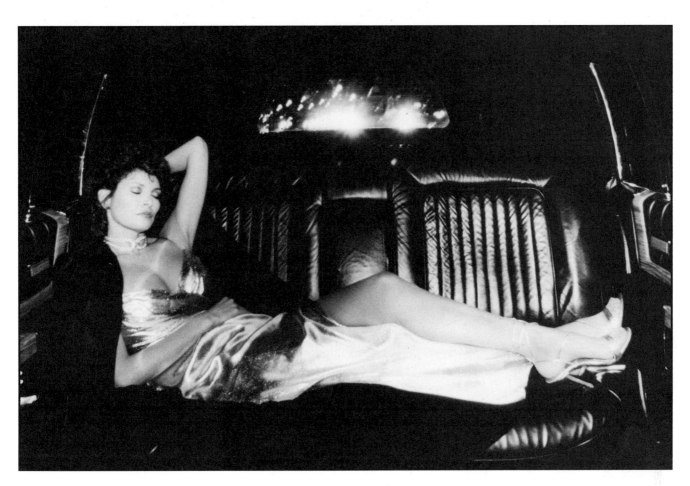

Above: *Demonstrating passive relaxation on the way back from the Palace Theatre each night.*

It's good to keep in mind that, although technological help is always welcome, it is only a copy of the original model—our body.

that allows you to function regularly at work or play with fewer recurring bouts of the same symptoms.

Active relaxation is the term I use to describe the way this series of yoga postures works. It's active, because you treat yourself and your distress by using rhythmic breathing and the systematic irrigation of fresh blood and oxygen to all parts of your body. It's relaxation, because you do so without adding any new distress in the process.

2. Organic Feedback

Electronic biofeedback is a technique that allows us to communicate better with our body by amplifying its impulses. But we already have our own built-in *organic feedback,* which does exactly the same thing. You will learn to develop, use, and understand it as part of this method.

It's good to keep in mind that, although technological help is always welcome, it is only a copy of the original model—our body. So you need not be totally dependent on outside help to fight distress symptoms when your best equipment is ultimately at your disposal.

Adapting the Method

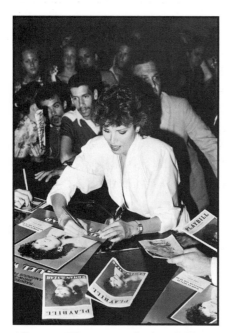

Above: *Not enough time? Even with a hectic schedule, one can always find time for the important things.*

First, you must decide that your *total* well-being is a priority worth the time and effort spent learning this program. Don't look around for loopholes or means of escape! With that in mind, I've listed some alternatives which may be useful *after,* and only after, you have completed the initial 30-to-60-day period and know the entire basic program. Please proceed with caution, however, if you're not an expert yet. Use your common sense—it should be in more plentiful supply now that you've been initiated into this method.

Not Enough Time

For those of you who have a particularly demanding schedule and find yourselves in a pinch, or never have enough time, the following three routines—while not suggested as an alternative to the entire basic program—will nonetheless provide you with the essentials, or at least maintain and keep your body toned until you find time again for a complete set.

Half-Series (40 to 45 minutes)

Simply do each of the poses *once,* instead of twice, in the exact same sequence. This series will provide you with the basic benefits of the program, but will not allow you to make the same degree of progress.

For beginners, it's only useful as a stopgap and shouldn't take the place of the full series in the initiation period of the first 30 to 60 days.

Mini-Series (25 to 30 minutes)

This abbreviated sequence will still bring you most of the benefits of the program, but should serve you as a "maintenance only" routine until you can switch back to the Half-Series or the complete set.

Perform each of the following postures twice:

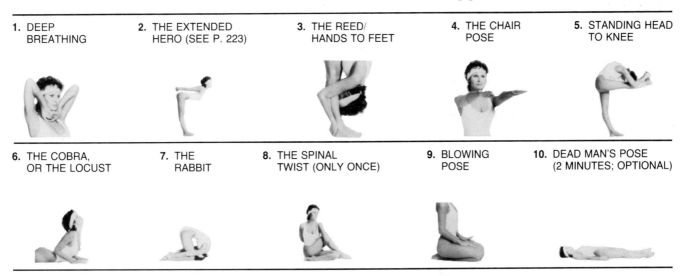

1. DEEP BREATHING
2. THE EXTENDED HERO (SEE P. 223)
3. THE REED/ HANDS TO FEET
4. THE CHAIR POSE
5. STANDING HEAD TO KNEE

6. THE COBRA, OR THE LOCUST
7. THE RABBIT
8. THE SPINAL TWIST (ONLY ONCE)
9. BLOWING POSE
10. DEAD MAN'S POSE (2 MINUTES; OPTIONAL)

Micro-Series (10 to 15 minutes)

When you're in a pinch and you need a quick boost—or just a welcome break in the middle of the day—the following will allow you to relieve tension, help you relax and concentrate better, and bring you fresh new energy and vitality. This is "instant yoga," but it's not as good as the real thing!

Note: Please do not force the muscles as hard as you would in a full series—this Micro-Series is a refresher, not a workout.

The following postures should be performed twice, except as noted:

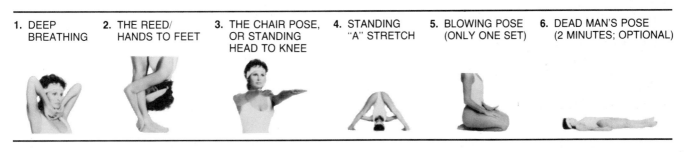

1. DEEP BREATHING
2. THE REED/ HANDS TO FEET
3. THE CHAIR POSE, OR STANDING HEAD TO KNEE
4. STANDING "A" STRETCH
5. BLOWING POSE (ONLY ONE SET)
6. DEAD MAN'S POSE (2 MINUTES; OPTIONAL)

Shortcuts

It's often handy to find a shortcut around the nonessentials, which vary from person to person. For example, I make these cuts when I'm pressed. Since I'm flexible and need more work on strength, I *always* do two sets of the standing postures. Then, if I have time, I include four floor postures: Cobra, Locust, Full Locust, and Bow, because they are very good for the derriere. Next I cut straight to the Rabbit to counteract all the back-bending, go to the Spinal Twist and the Blowing Pose, and then I'm done. Once you know the routine, you can invent your own shortcuts.

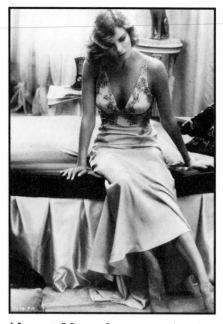

Above: *My wake-up routine in the film* The Wild Party. *Make your approach to each day a nonviolent one.*

Waking up doesn't have to consist of pouring coffee down your gullet to shock yourself into the day.

Wake-up Routine

When I wake up every morning, I roll right out of bed and onto a mat I placed on the floor the night before. The hard surface feels so good, even after sleeping on a firm mattress, that I'm able to release any last tension that has unconsciously settled in my body during the night. Sometimes I do the Knee Squeeze with a pillow tucked under my hips—it's good for the lower back.

Then, I raise my legs without tension into the air, to start the blood flowing. I stay like that until I feel my head clear, then I get up and take a moment to drop down over my legs and hang there like a dead weight, allowing my hamstrings to release. Sometimes I like to clasp my arms behind my back—as in the Extended Hero—to relax tension in the neck and shoulders. Other times, I clasp my elbows in front of me. The extra body weight helps to free the hips and lower back. Finally, I take a shower and finish my morning ritual.

This is my routine for waking up. You can judge for yourself what's best for you. If you're a morning enthusiast, it sets you up wonderfully for the exercise later. Once you have started practicing this method regularly, you can devise your own morning routine to satisfy your individual needs.

I offer this only to suggest that waking up doesn't have to consist of pouring coffee down your gullet to shock yourself into the day. I've learned to prefer a smooth transition from one activity into the next, instead of piling up an array of small violences against myself from the moment I wake up. As you are no doubt aware, we treat others much the way we treat ourselves. Don't be ruthless with yourself and you won't be with others. I think your attitude to the outside world is a reflection of your attitude toward yourself. You know I'm right.

Once you become aware of the harmony in your body, you will also become more acutely attuned to the menace of disharmony in your life-style, your eating habits, your relationships with other people, and even the atmosphere—such as the weather, or any psychological depression in and around you. The ability to compensate in these areas, to even out the imbalances and make things flow, will come to you naturally. Eventually you will be able to accommodate your own life to your personal needs.

It doesn't really matter what motivated you to open the door to this method. The residual effects come right along with the physical culture. I cannot emphasize enough that, whatever your goal is, it is the approach to it that counts.

Join me, and make your approach to each day a nonviolent one.

Special Postures for Special People

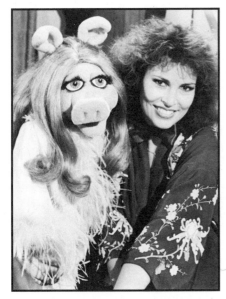

Above: *Being a living legend has its price—Miss Piggy confided that she too suffers from tension headaches.*

What makes this method different is that it deals with emotional stress as well as the physical side of fitness. Stress levels are often the most difficult to overcome, and they really do stand in the way of your performance as an individual, on the job, and in the business world.

Executive Stress

Stress is so common today, among executives and professionals in all walks of life, that it's reached epidemic proportions. So, it is to those unsung heroes that this section is dedicated. To every "desk jockey"—big shot or not—who labors unflinchingly on the phone for hours until it almost becomes an appendage. To the dedicated perfectionist who is imprisoned in an office after hours. And even to the diligent bureaucrat who is shackled by red tape, but plunges ahead in spite of it.

Pain in the Neck

The following pages are not meant to replace the entire series, but only to augment it. They zero in on that favorite area of tension—around the neck and shoulders—which causes so many headaches and stiff necks, as well as irritability. The problem with a pain in the neck is that it keeps coming back to plague you again and again. It is therefore helpful to know these postures—not just to relieve the pain, but to ward it off when you first feel it coming on. Get up from your desk, close the door to your office, and do them.

The Writer's Pose

The Writer's Pose came in handy when I was writing this book. Anyone who must sit hunched over a desk for long periods of time (students, secretaries, bookkeepers, Presidents of the U.S., etc.) is susceptible to tightness and muscle spasms that settle in the shoulders and scapulae. This pose will be helpful to them.

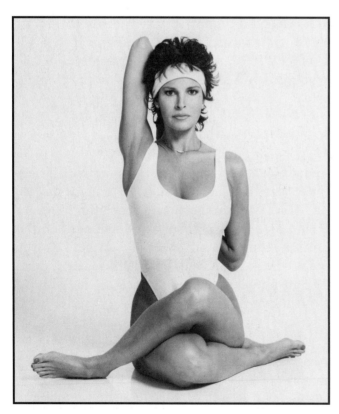 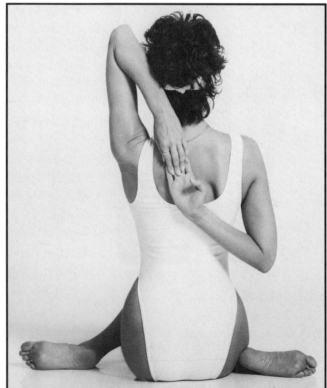

1. Sit on both hips evenly, your legs bent back, one knee on top of the other. Reach over your shoulder with the opposite arm to the top leg. Now, bend the other arm around to the back, as though you had to scratch, and overlap your fingertips. Then, pull *up* with the top arm and *down* with the bottom arm. Hold for 20 seconds and breathe normally.

2. This is the rear view, so that you can see the exact grip. Keep the hips even on the floor and your head as straight as possible. When you're finished with 20 counts, release the hands and REPEAT on the other side. If your hands won't touch behind your back, grab a dish towel or the like and play tug-of-war with that. This pose can also be done in a chair or standing.

The Extended Hero

I like to call this pose the Overextended Hero, because that's what it seems the modern businessman has become. Each day looms as a battle—a campaign against the odds of the stock market, interest rates, the board of directors, office politics, and the demands of family. They all crawl up the back of your neck and gather there for the attack.

So, upon awaking or any other time, when they start to come in for the kill, try this pose.

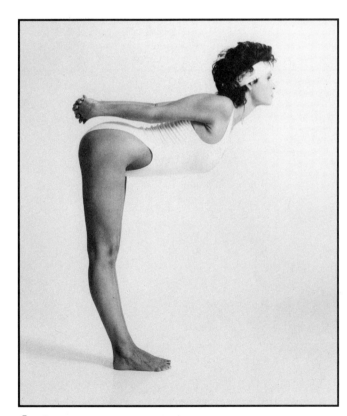

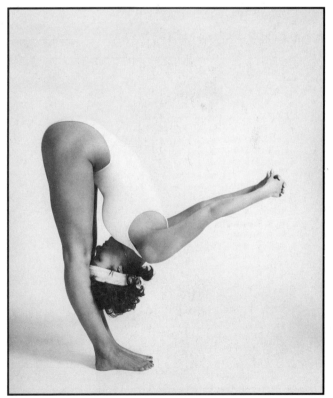

1. Stand up straight, feet together, knees locked. Clasp your hands behind your back, fingers interlaced. Inhale, expanding the chest and pulling back the shoulders.

On the exhale, start bending forward from the hips with the back straight, head up at first, bottom stuck out. Keep your weight resting on the heels.

2. Continue forward slowly, and drop your head toward your legs. Lift the arms up and away from your body.

If you can get down this far, curl your chin in and drop your forehead to the knees. *Do not force it.* Hold for a few moments. Concentrate on exhalation. Inhale and come up *slowly.* This pose can also be done in a kneeling position by placing your forehead on the floor in front of your knees.

The Survivor

This pose is an alternative to the Standing "A" Head to Knee; I discovered it when I suffered a severe muscle spasm in my neck caused by too much anxiety and tension, which seemed impossible to relieve. The Survivor helps eliminate the pull on the trapezius muscles, which run between your shoulder blades and up both sides of your neck. When, after one of "those days," your shoulders feel like they're up around your ears, try this pose. It really works!

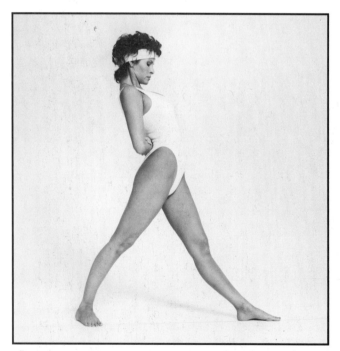

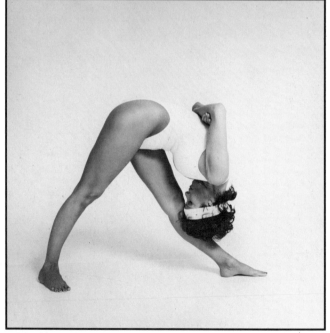

1. Stand with your feet wide apart, hands together over your head. Turn one foot to the side and then swivel your hips and the upper body to face in the same direction. Inhale.

Clasp your hands behind your back, in the same manner as you would fold them across your chest. The forearms should be rotated slightly and the hands should hold the inside of the arms. Tuck your chin in.

2. Inhale and go forward from the hips. Aim for the knee, keeping your chin tucked *in* and curving your spine inward. Stay there for 10 counts and come up slowly. If your head won't go to the knee, bend the knee up to meet the forehead, or do the best you can. This puts more attention on the neck than the shoulders, and is good for the trapezius area that knots so easily under tension.

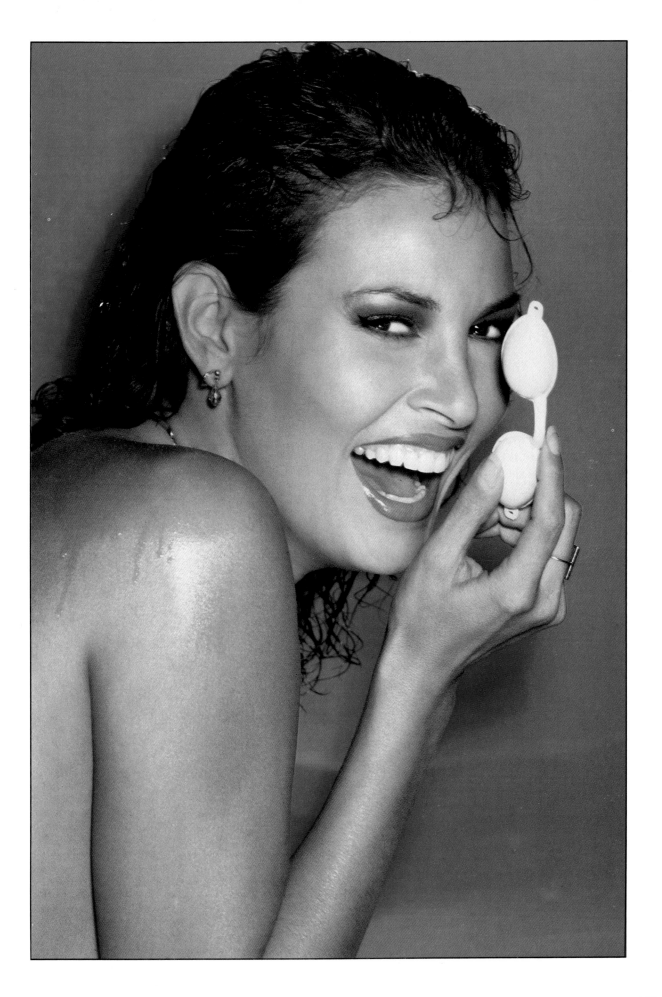

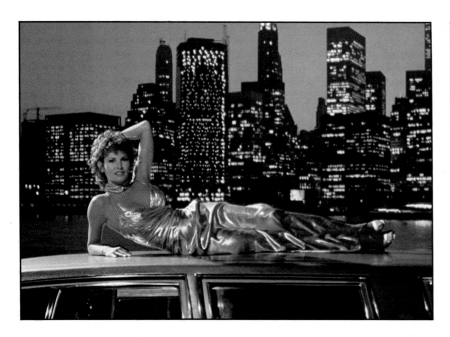

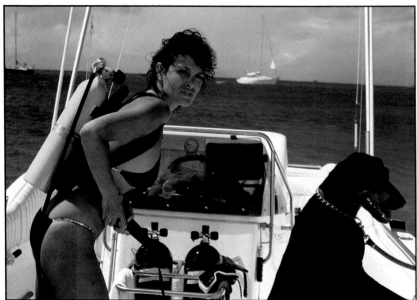

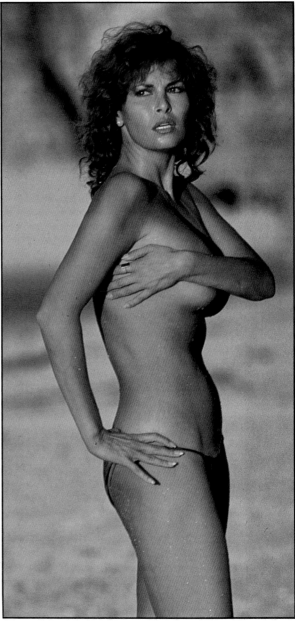

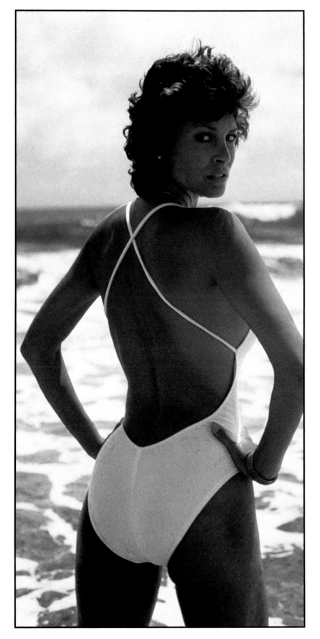

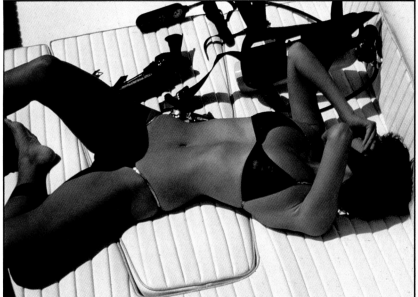

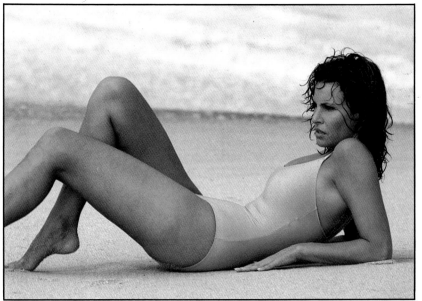

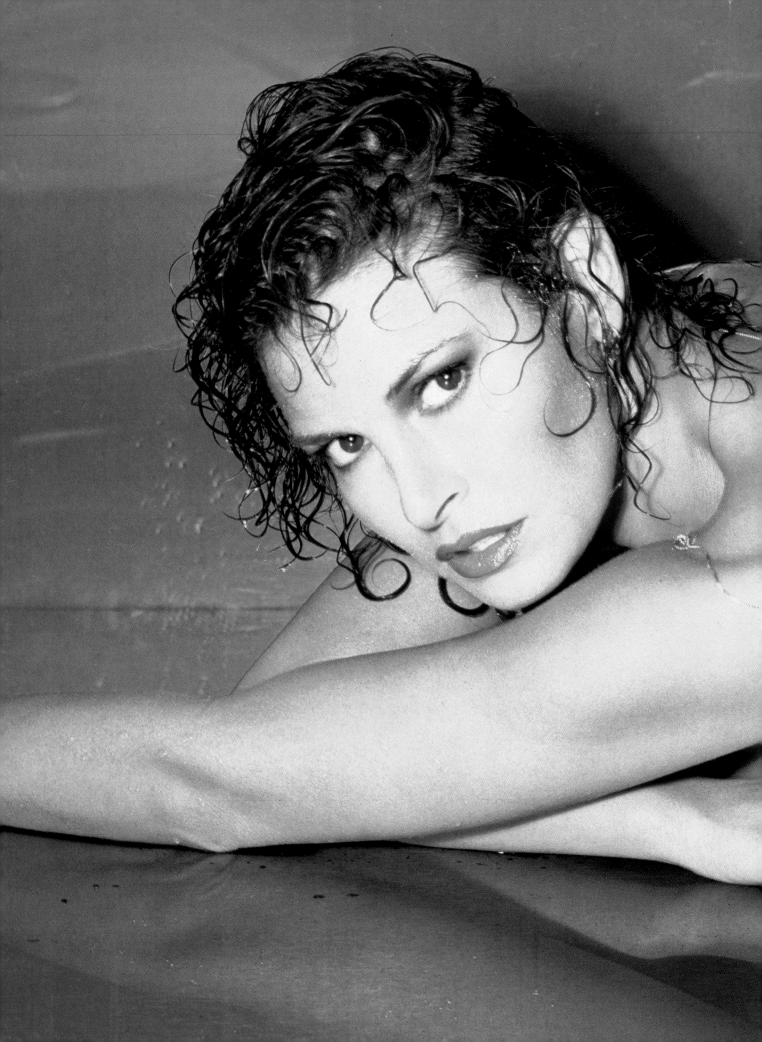

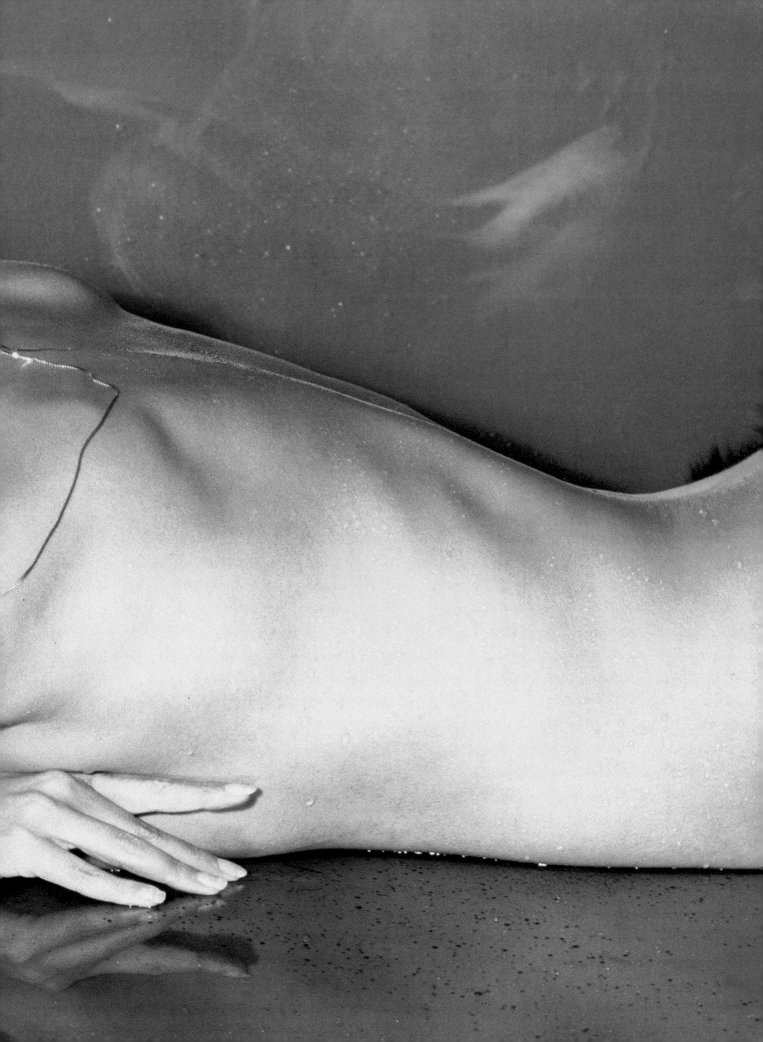

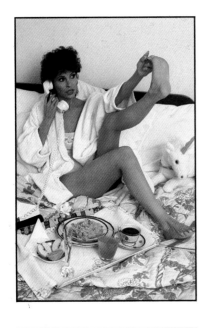

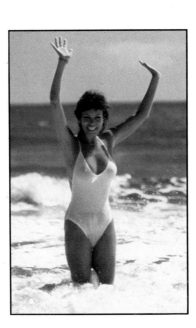

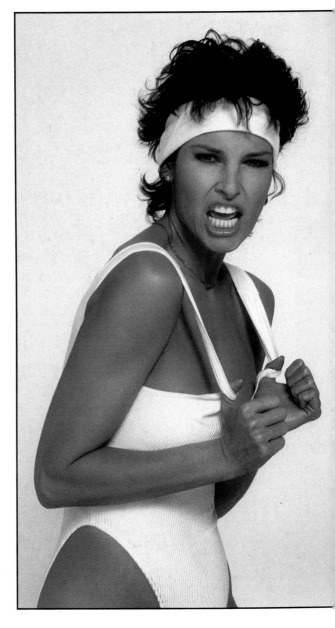

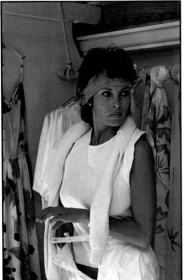

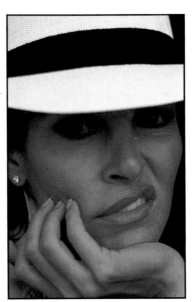

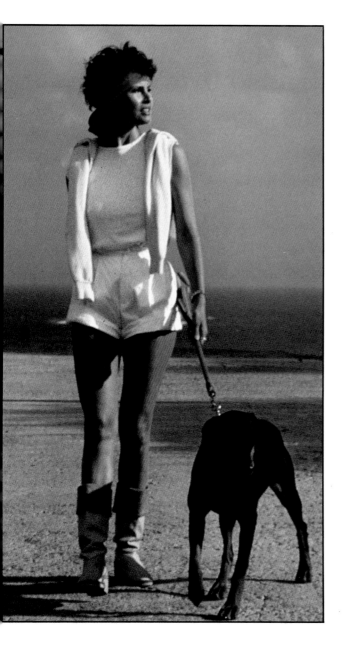

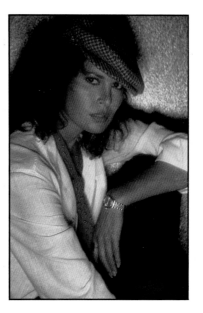

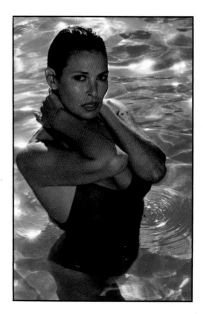

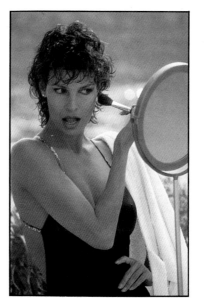

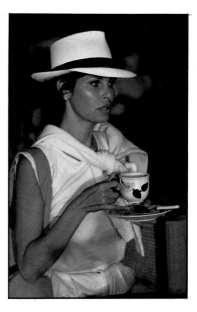

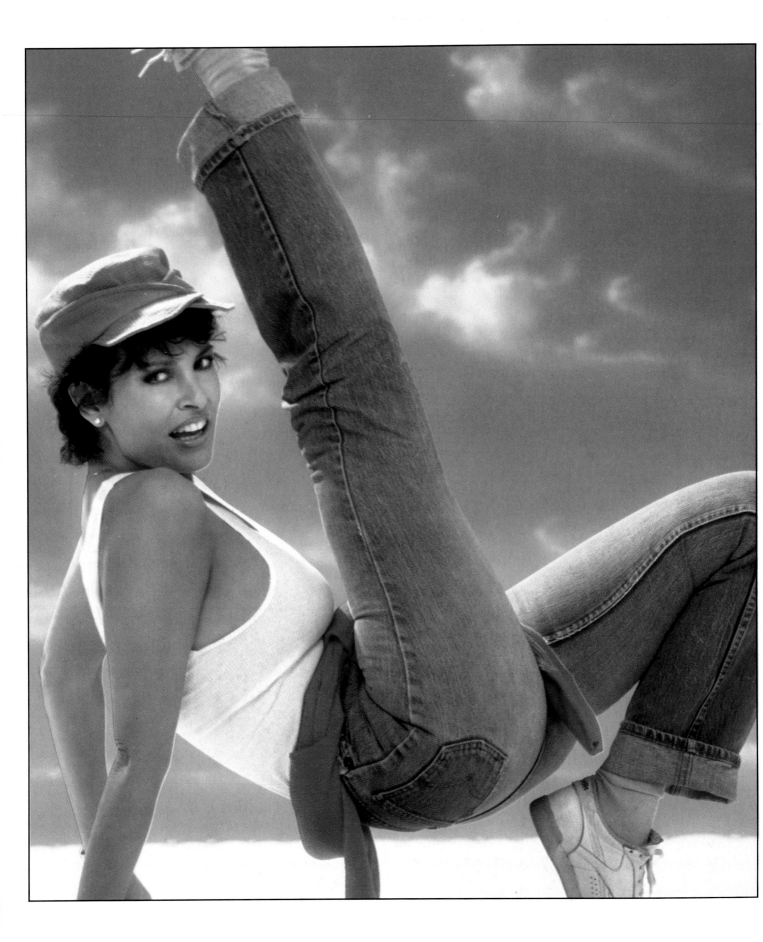

Food for Thought

Human beings are the only creatures that live to eat rather than eat to live.

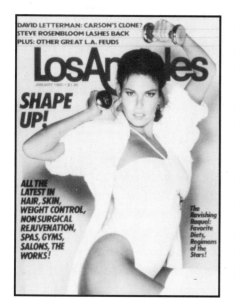

One of the most exciting rewards of this method is that you will end up becoming your own best nutritionist. You actually begin to develop a built-in radar system that determines what food your body needs and what it doesn't.

This doesn't mean that you'll be a member of the fruit-and-nuts group. On the contrary, a well-functioning body is always happy to extract any energy it can from any food. But, needless to say, once you've got your body all streamlined and purring away like a well-oiled machine, you'll become about as finicky about its care and feeding as a bachelor with a shiny new Ferrari. Junk food will automatically be *out*.

Nutritional Nirvana

Human beings are the only creatures that live to eat rather than eat to live. Personally, I love to eat; but in the profession I've chosen, it would be catastrophic if I ate everything for fun and flavor. I'd overeat like crazy! I prefer to get my fun and flavor from my style of life. So I have to guard against overindulgence at the dinner table. Fortunately, my daily yoga practice gives me plenty of energy and discipline to resist, and I find that I'm not so easily tempted.

When your digestion is operating inefficiently, chances are that for every pound of food you eat, you're capable of absorbing only 25 percent of the nutrients it has to offer. The rest, which is waste, cannot be eliminated properly, so it stays in your body, forming toxins. In effect, you are making your own toxicity, plus fat and cholesterol, causing high blood pressure, heart trouble, and fatigue.

As you progress in this yoga program, you will be able to

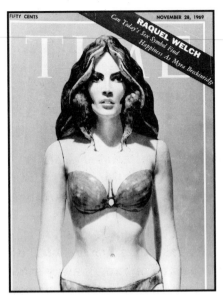

absorb more nutrients from the food you eat. Thus you will gradually need less food to fuel your energy, and less of your intake will stay in your body as waste, to pollute the tissues and exhaust the system. You will also find you need less sleep. Oversleep is often just a crutch your body needs when your digestive system is overloaded or working poorly. I used to need 8 to 10 hours of sleep a night, now I never need more than 6.

I've learned that eating right involves three elements:

1. Where you eat

2. How you eat

3. What you eat

This sequence is important, because by the time the food is in your mouth and on its way to your stomach, there's not much you can do about it. So I believe it's the approach to eating that counts.

Where You Eat

Is the place where you eat noisy, "overstimulating"? Is it ugly, drab, depressing? Does the service remind you of Jack Nicholson's restaurant scene in *Five Easy Pieces*? All these things can and do affect your digestion and the ability to assimilate nutrients from your food. Emotional relaxation is much more important to digestion than it is usually given credit for. And to make matters worse, anxiety and depression contribute immeasurably to gaining weight.

I try to eat in an atmosphere of calm and good service, even if that means eating something first before meeting friends.

I try to eat in an atmosphere of calm and good service, even if that means eating something first before meeting friends. The frenzy involved in certain social or business occasions where food is served as a formality is so unsettling that it gives me indigestion from just thinking about it. Don't show up hungry: eat a snack beforehand. Then you won't be tempted to eat badly and consume too much alcohol.

How You Eat

As we race through our modern lives, if we want to sustain the speed that is almost sacred to our American way of life, we end up with less and less time to eat. As a result, a new phenomenon has surfaced in our eating habits. You've heard of speed reading—just the high points, none of the substance? Now we have "speed eating"—just the taste, none of the essentials. I've never been a big speed freak myself. Haste makes waste is my motto. The Chinese have a proverb: "Drink what you eat and eat what

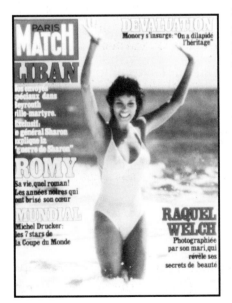

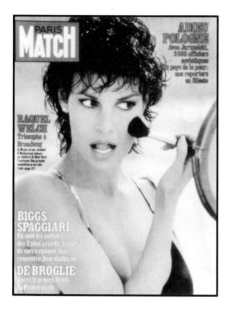

you drink," which in simple English means, Take the time to chew *and* swallow.

For example while talking energetically over a meal, chances are you're gulping air and swallowing your food nearly whole, like the shark in *Jaws II*. The only problem is, your stomach doesn't possess the same enzymes as a shark's. So the food, especially red meat, just sits there like dead weight until your body can assimilate it.

Eating too fast is sometimes just a case of being overhungry. When I get involved in my work, I don't even think about food until my stomach sends up danger signals—and then look out! When I'm ravenous, I could eat roof shingles whole!

To avoid these little hunger attacks, I take along snacks to munch on all day. I pack fruit and rice cakes or a small container of brown rice—just a spoonful keeps the wolf of hunger away from my door. I hate to go to a restaurant ravenous; it makes me eat all the bread on the table and puts me in a ferocious mood.

To sum up, eat less food, but at more frequent intervals, and *slow down* when you eat!

What You Eat

If you've chosen an overactive—some say "colorful"—life, as I have, you have to offset it with your diet. Forget about eating ten-course meals like an eighteenth-century marquise. Even if your pocketbook can afford it, your waistline can't.

I know, I know, the Europeans can get away with it! But quite frankly, their food is of better quality and more often organically grown, without chemicals and hothouse techniques. Also, stress levels are lower, since the structure of their societies allows a longer break in the business day to enjoy eating, to relax and converse. Their priorities are different. Many Europeans gain weight when they come to this country because of the food, the eating habits, and the pace.

It is said that the Europeans know the art of living, while we Americans have mastered the art of making money. Perhaps we'd both do well to learn something from each other. In the meantime, my advice is to streamline yourself and your eating habits for the twenty-first century. Now is the time to start!

What to eat and what not to eat, that is the question—and it's got us up to our eyeballs in trends.

My Eating Basics

Even though thousands of women have asked me about my diet, when I tell them, most are unprepared for the answer. When

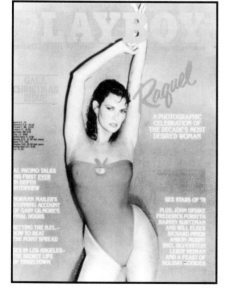

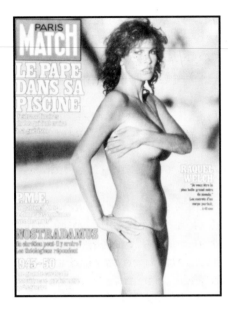

I get all the flavor and excitement I need from my life and work, so I don't need as much "pizzazz" from my food.

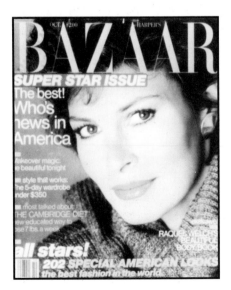

they hear that in addition to the routine offered in this book I have given up salt, sugar, oil, processed food and refined grains and breads, and certain dairy products, they are aghast. They protest that they could never go through such torture.

The truth is, I have a very sensitive stomach and have been on a rather restrictive diet for the last several years. On top of which, I am a Virgo; we Virgos are said to have an overactive mind and our mental gymnastics play havoc with our digestion. So, even though I have to be more careful than most people about what I eat, I've taken the point of view that I get all the flavor and excitement I need from my life and work. So I don't need as much "pizzazz" from my food.

For years I ignored the advice of doctors who wanted to put me on a strict diet, but my stomach caught up with me and I had to change. I think I resisted because I've never had a real weight problem, but then I never felt really 100 percent either. So now I have knuckled under to a new way of eating and am much better off. I don't suffer bloating and painful indigestion; and those stubborn areas of fat that used to linger on my hips and abdomen have disappeared. You don't have to be overweight to have these problems—eating the wrong things can cause them as well.

I can't recommend what I eat for everyone, but I can assure you that the basic approach to good eating is the same for most people. I advise that everyone consult a doctor or nutritionist about a special custom-made diet.

When I first sought nutritional advice on my own, I was inundated by what I heard in the locker rooms of various health clubs and exercise classes. Everyone had a diet and everyone seemed confused. Quite frankly, I think the subject was a bit overworked because merely *talking* about diets convinced most of us that we were actually *on* one.

Often, we'd exchange "finds" with one another until it seemed that every exotic possibility had been explored. There was talk of fantastic doctors with placenta injections, a new diet book that had you eating nothing but papaya for months on end; each new tidbit was absolutely fascinating. Finally, after exploring a few of these ideas and finding myself not all that fond of papayas, I stumbled upon a bona fide nutritionist who put me on a comprehensive plan to fit my body, my emotional needs, and my professional life.

Good Nutrition

I have since learned that good nutrition is not a diet or a short-term measure, it's a way of life. So no diet worth its (lack of) salt is something to jump into lightly, any more than you would jump

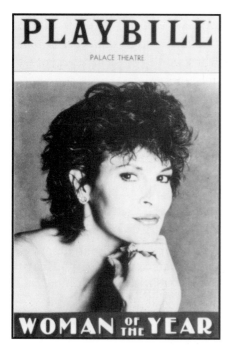

into a serious romance! It's important to understand that there are many factors, like blood type, body type, and life-style, that affect your digestion and the nutrients you need. Locker-room diets cannot provide for these variables, not even if they're borrowed from your best friend.

Certain general principles are common to most practical nutritional advice. They are designed to reeducate your taste buds, cleanse your entire digestive system, and pave the way for the reintroduction of certain foods (not all foods) into your diet according to your individual needs.

If you're under thirty, adopting these guidelines will form good habits now, so you won't have a lot of remedial work later. For those of you who, over the years, have already fallen into bad habits—and I'm one of them!—it will take time to readjust. In either case, a healthy diet can help you drop unwanted pounds, unlock energy, alert your senses, and gain mental clarity.

Keep in mind that *diet alone is not enough*. A combination of diet, exercise, and environment ensure that your good health and beauty will stand the test of time.

Finally, it's worth repeating, that if you've already been practicing this method of exercise for a while (for 30 days or more), you'll be ahead of the game: the adjustment will be easier. Okay, everyone, are you ready?

Vitamin Supplements

Finally, if our food were all organically grown and our livestock not force-fed, if there were less use of pesticides and hothouse techniques, we would be able to get full value from the food we eat. But with today's farming methods and the stress levels that affect modern society, vitamin supplements are essential. They ensure that we get the nutrients that are missing from our food or that we do not assimilate because of nervous tension.

I take daily doses of:

● Vitamin C
● Vitamin B Complex
● Vitamin E with Selenium
● Calcium with Vitamin D
● Multivitamin Tablets

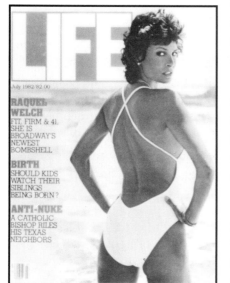

To be assimilated effectively, vitamins should be taken after meals. Take at least the daily dosage listed, except in the cases of vitamins A, D, E, and K. These vitamins have been known to cause side effects if taken in excess. So consult your doctor for recommendations.

Nutritional Guidelines

1. No-Nos

No Salt
No Sugar
No Caffeine
No Oil, or use very sparingly
No Preservatives

If you're alarmed at the idea that no extra salt, oil, or sugar is needed in our diet, remember that *they are already present in our natural foods* without having to add them.

By cutting out these unnecessary additives you will reawaken your taste buds and begin to appreciate the tangy natural flavor of undoctored food. It's like breaking a drug habit. A couple of weeks of "cold turkey," and you won't even miss them!

Cutting out salt can reduce the fluid retention that so many women suffer from. Your body will become less puffy. I even found it helped in reducing swelling in my face and around my eyes.

As for caffeine, it's a stimulant—it kicks your adrenals into action, even when they are tired and run-down. My nutritionist, Eileen Poole, equates it to "beating a dead horse."

2. Protein

Chicken and Turkey: Yes
Fish: Yes
Veal: Yes
Red Meat: Sometimes (once a week). Lamb and liver are best (calf's liver is better, if you can afford it!).
Eggs are sometimes hard to digest for some people.

I eat mostly chicken, fish, and veal because they are easier for me to digest. Anything that makes your digestion run smoothly will help you lose weight. Don't bog down your system with heavier foods that take more time and energy to assimilate. I usually eat only ¼ pound of protein a meal to leave room for a large portion of vegetables.

When I am engaged in strenuous activity, like dancing and singing, as I did on Broadway in the musical *Woman of the Year*, I add more protein to my diet. Then I eat lamb and liver more often, and occasionally beef. Your own intake of red meat depends on how athletic you are and also, of course, on your doctor's advice.

3. Vegetables

Green Vegetables: Yes. Cooked veggies, preferably steamed, are easier to digest if you have problems with gas and bloating.
Zucchini
Green Beans
Artichoke
Asparagus
Spinach
Summer/Yellow Squash
Broccoli
Chinese Pea Pods
Parsley
Celery
Potatoes: Yes. If combined with a green vegetable instead of a protein (see Food Combining, page 241).
Root Vegetables: Yes. Carrots, turnips, beets, etc.

The vegetables listed above are the ones I concentrate on in my diet because they're high in nutritional value and easier to digest. However, some people can tolerate a wider selection, including eggplant, green peas, leeks, mushrooms, cauliflower, tomatoes, and many others.

Vegetables contain important vitamins, minerals, and nutrients that your body needs. You cannot get these in salads alone. I make it a point to eat vegetables twice a day with protein—it aids in digesting the protein and cleanses the system.

4. Salads

Romaine: Yes
Boston Bibb Lettuce: Yes

Be aware that iceberg lettuce, which is part of the cabbage family, can cause gastritis and bloating in some people. I choose to stay away from it, even though it's the kind we usually find in most restaurant salad bowls.

I've adopted the French habit of eating salad at the end of a meal, *after the main course*. It cleans the palate and is a better aid to digestion when eaten last. In matters of food, the French have got it down to a fine art.

5. Fruits

Fruit: Yes. Cooked is easier to digest; avoid canned fruit if possible, but if you use it *always rinse the syrup off first*. 2 fruits daily provide enough natural-sugar intake. *Count one fruit juice as one whole fruit*.

I always dilute my fruit juices with water, half and half. It really helps to cut down the sugar intake. If you are interested in losing weight, remember that fruit is a great source of natural sugar—but don't overdo it.

6. Whole Grains

Whole Grains: Yes. Wheat is sometimes a problem for people with allergies, asthma, and breathing and sinus problems.

I eat oatmeal or cooked grain without milk or salt for breakfast, because dairy products don't agree with me. For sugar, I top it off with slices of baked apple, pear, or peach and sprinkle with a dash of cinnamon.

Bread: *Keep to a minimum*. Toast is better and easier to digest. I never eat hot dough fresh from the oven. It's delicious, but you should avoid it, unless you find it amusing to swell up like a blimp.

I always carry around rye crackers and rice cakes as snacks. Some people refer to them as "air cakes," but they are filling and soothing when you're past mealtime. They also keep you from grabbing a candy bar instead!

Nutritional Guidelines

7. Dairy Products

Dairy products are okay for most people, although they may present a problem for those suffering from allergies, sinus congestion, asthma, breathing difficulty, and indigestion.

Milk, Cheese, Butter, Yogurt: Yes, but don't overindulge.

I have cut out all dairy products in the last few years, but I don't recommend that for everyone. I stay away for two reasons: they congest the lymphatic system and cause phlegm, which inhibits the use of my voice as a singer and actress.

A little milk used occasionally in cooking, a little cheese, unsalted butter, or yogurt is alright. But use them sparingly, and get your doctor's advice. By the way, hard, nonprocessed cheese is usually easier to digest than soft cheese spreads.

8. Cooking Methods

Steamed: Yes
Broiled: Yes
Grilled: Yes
Poached: Yes
Fried, Sautéed, or Sauced: Who are you kidding?

For seasoning, I use lemon and herbs or sometimes unsalted mustard.

When I am dining at a restaurant, I always ask for steamed vegetables and broiled, grilled, or poached protein. It seems that the better the restaurant, the more gracious and willing they are to oblige. If the menu shows the entrees with a sauce, I ask for my sauce on the side.

When I am invited to a dinner party, I usually eat first before I go!

9. Drinking

Water: Yes
Fresh Fruit Juices: Yes
Wine: Only occasionally, and preferably diluted half and half with water, like fruit juice. (I know, it's sacrilege.)

All in all, I recommend 6–8 glasses of water a day. I drink a glass of water:

1. First thing in the morning

2. Last thing before bed

3. Never with meals—it dilutes the digestive juices

4. At least a half hour after eating, or in between meals.

Note: Room temperature or warm is best for most drinks. Break the ice habit!

Lemon water: helpful for those losing weight or cleansing the system from illness, colds, or virus. It's a great source of vitamin C and it can also relieve constipation.

I admit that these Nutritional Guidelines are tough, and that you may feel like you're eating cardboard in the beginning. But I found that after the first two "death defying" weeks I was home free!

Food-Combining

Any good cook knows that combining ingredients makes all the difference. The same thing applies in the recipe for total health and beauty. Food combining is merely the principle of what foods go together, to aid better digestion and weight loss.

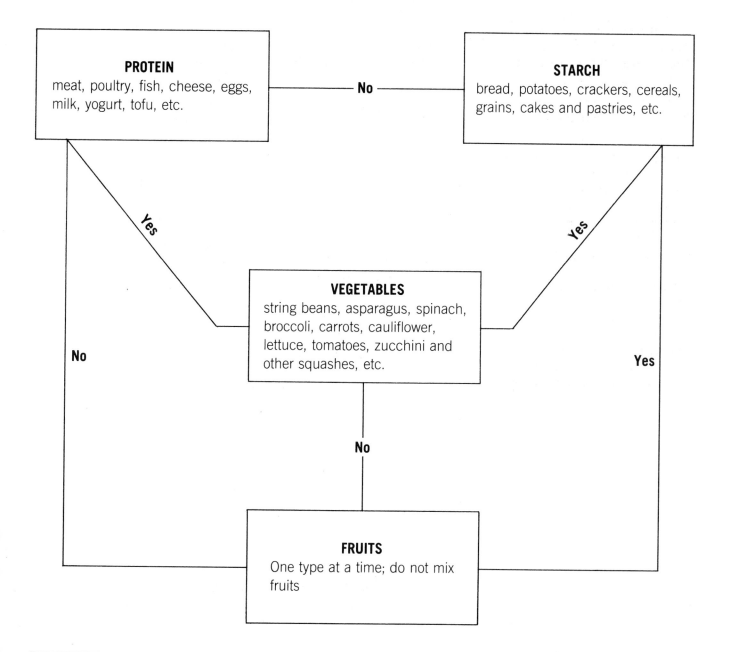

PROTEIN
meat, poultry, fish, cheese, eggs, milk, yogurt, tofu, etc.

— No —

STARCH
bread, potatoes, crackers, cereals, grains, cakes and pastries, etc.

Yes

Yes

VEGETABLES
string beans, asparagus, spinach, broccoli, carrots, cauliflower, lettuce, tomatoes, zucchini and other squashes, etc.

No

Yes

No

FRUITS
One type at a time; do not mix fruits

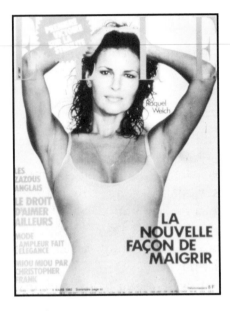

I've been known to devour an entire apple pie at a single sitting. I just can't stand the thought of the pie sitting there uneaten all night long.

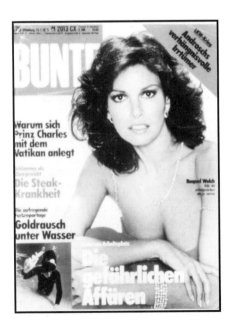

Food Combining

Midriff bulge and saddlebag hips will be on their way out if you follow food-combining principles. But diet alone will not do it. You should combine good eating habits with this daily exercise routine. That way you reinforce your gains on both fronts. There are only two main rules.

RULE 1: DO NOT EAT PROTEIN AND STARCH TOGETHER AT THE SAME MEAL.

For example: If you decide on pasta, just eat it with vegetables—skip the meat or fish—and make sure to eat *equal amounts* of vegetable and pasta. The other option is to decide on meat or another protein for the main course, in which case skip the potatoes, and bring on that equal portion of vegetables again. Simple, no?

RULE 2: DO NOT EAT FRUIT WITH VEGETABLES OR PROTEIN AT THE SAME MEAL.

An exception to this rule is apples, for some people. Eat fruit separately (try to wait at least a half hour after a meal) or as a snack between meals. It is alright to eat fruit with some starches, such as on your morning cereal. In fact, it's better than using sugar.

This simple chart covers the basic food-combining principles. Generally speaking, you can't go wrong by following this guide. Special exceptions to the rule are best prescribed by a doctor or qualified nutritionist.

Cheating

People always ask me if I ever break down. Does my ironclad willpower ever falter? Well, everyone cheats from time to time. I hate to admit it, but I've been known to devour an entire apple pie at a single sitting. I just can't stand the thought of the pie sitting there uneaten all night long. It haunts my dreams! But usually I'm very disciplined. For example, I stayed religiously on my prescribed diet for three years before straying from the fold. It must be some kind of a record, but it really wasn't much of a sacrifice. Once I had reeducated my taste buds, I started to discover the natural flavor of food for the first time.

Usually, after the first few weeks of any diet, the urge to cheat is gone. Getting off to a good start is everything: just like a rocket to the moon, once you're launched, you're on your way.

I could never, never encourage you to be casual about your own nutritional plan. But if you should fall by the wayside and happen to sneak a side order of french fries or maybe a piece of

THE WONDER SOUP

1 qt. water
1 lb. string beans, strings removed
2 or 3 celery stalks, strings removed, chopped
1 bunch parsley, stems removed, finely chopped
3 or 4 zucchini, chopped

In a deep saucepan, bring a quart of water to a boil. Place string beans, celery, and parsley in water and let boil for 5 minutes. Add the zucchini and continue boiling for another 3 to 4 minutes.

Remove vegetables from water with a slotted spoon (save the water). Puree them in a blender. Use the cooking water to thin the puree to the desired thickness. The consistency of pea soup is usually the best.

The best way to get rid of any remaining strings from the celery and beans is to first Puree, then Grind, and finally Blend in a blender.

Note: Some people cannot eat zucchini. Check with your doctor and/or nutritionist.

chocolate cake for dessert, you may need help getting back on track.

So here's a solution I use to avoid getting discouraged and falling still further into an eating binge. It's a green vegetable soup . . . that I call the "Wonder Soup."

The Wonder Soup

This special soup is a lifesaver, the best homemade remedy I've found since old-fashioned chicken soup. Trumpets and fanfare would be but faint praise for the all-time great green Wonder Soup. Unfortunately, it looks like something from *The Exorcist*. Maybe that's not a coincidence, because if something ails you, here comes this green remedy to save the day!

The Wonder Soup *equalizes* your system and helps to *cleanse away* all of your transgressions. In addition, anytime you feel low, sluggish, or run-down and on the verge of catching something, it's an excellent remedy. I always take it to ward off colds or the flu, and I haven't had a dose of antibiotics in over three years!

Although this is not a gourmet treat, I've come to enjoy the subtle flavor of this saltless soup. When you see how healthy you look and feel, it begins to taste pretty good. Sometimes, if I've had a rough night, I even eat it for breakfast!

Nutritionists: A New Breed

There are so many factors that affect each of us differently— and thus our digestion, and the nutrients we need—that no formula diet can work for everyone.

I've tried here to give you the basics of good nutrition, and perhaps some tips that will help you. But I know from experience that a good nutritionist can do wonders to guide you into good eating habits, whether it's for weight loss or health reasons. Food has mental and physical dimensions, too. A balanced diet will help you on both fronts.

For most of my life I ate what everyone else was eating, and thought that if I didn't feel good there must be something wrong with *me*. Years later, I realized that I was different, and after consulting a nutritionist learned to eat what was right for me.

Like many other Americans, I ate junk food as a teenager. But when I became pregnant with my first child at nineteen, I quickly cleaned up my act: I became very careful about what I ate, but it still wasn't enough.

I was under pressure. I was young and slightly terrified of having a baby. I was also doing a morning television show, a sort

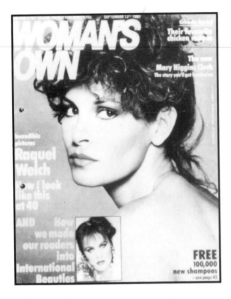

Nutritionists were people who planned school lunches at the campus cafeteria. They decided whether it was going to be tacos and beans, or Salisbury steak and mashed potatoes. Thank God those days are gone.

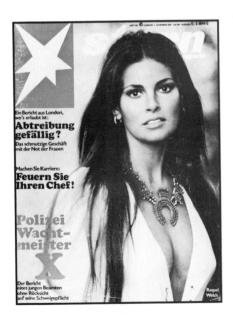

of "Good Morning America" on a local channel in San Diego. I did the weather and occasional interviews, and had to rise and shine very early every morning. But it never occurred to me that this kind of schedule, plus the wear and tear on my nerves, would affect my digestion.

I used to wake up at 4:00 A.M. . . . throw up . . . try to eat . . . dress . . . do my makeup . . . drive to the studio . . . have a doughnut (that's all they had) . . . throw up . . . get my material off the AP and UPI wire services . . . try soda crackers . . . make my notes . . . and finally manage to smile and be bright-eyed and bushy-tailed on camera, after which I would once again . . . throw up!

I didn't know then that, in addition to morning sickness, I was allergic to wheat and had an overacidic stomach that reacted badly to raw food. I would have been better off if I'd been eating baby food *myself* while awaiting my baby.

Anyhow, I had a beautiful baby boy, Damon—7 pounds, 7 ounces—healthy and energetic. I gained only about 14 pounds during the pregnancy, with all the morning sickness, and recovered nicely. But I still didn't know what the problem was. So by the time I had my second child, a girl, Tahnee, about two years later, I think I held the record for morning nausea.

That was at a time when doctors didn't delve deeply into nutrition. Nutritionists were people who planned school lunches at the campus cafeteria. They decided whether it was going to be tacos and beans, or Salisbury steak and mashed potatoes. Thank God those days are gone.

I learned everything I know about my own eating requirements from my nutritionist, Eileen Poole. Until then it was trial and error. I've never been fat, so I'd never gone to a doctor to lose weight. But that's not the only criterion of good health. Your diet must give you energy and support the life-style you've chosen. It must circumvent the dangers of certain foods to your system. If you give it a chance to work, proper diet can help give you a feeling of tremendous well-being.

Doctors and psychotherapists are just beginning to recognize the correlation between diet and nervous disorders. But a nutritional approach is not a diet—it is a *way of life*. I've sent both of my children to nutritionists so that they can have the benefits of eating correctly, within their own individual guidelines.

Food Is Your Best Medicine

It's never been clear to me why the Western medical profession, with few exceptions, has been so slow to accept the empirical knowledge that there is a correlation between food and disease (both physical and mental). It's nothing new. On the contrary, it's

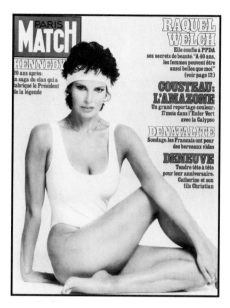

fundamental. Perhaps we've all been somewhat seduced by the rather remarkable strides made in pharmaceuticals (drugs) and surgery. But that shouldn't take precedence over what we know to be organically sound—namely, that good nutrition is the best preventive medicine. If you abuse your body through improper diet (what is improper for you), it will pave the way for diseases of every variety, from cancer to heart disease and emphysema. An excellent book on this subject is *Food Is Your Best Medicine,* by Henry G. Bieler.

Just recently, I received a bulletin from the American Institute for Cancer Research, for which I served as honorary chairman in 1975. In it was the following statement: "Breast cancer may be *prevented* and perhaps even *controlled* through proper diet. Experts now estimate that 60 percent of the cancer in women may be *caused* by the wrong diet." I am not surprised.

It stands to reason that, if improper diet can create a toxic climate in the body that invites disease, the reverse is also true. That same disease can be cured or controlled by the proper use of the correct foods. Surely the use of drugs and surgery should come into play only as a last resort. No surgeon is anxious to perform unnecessary and risky procedures, or prescribe drugs, with their accompanying side effects, before all other avenues have been explored. But it is also true that not enough doctors are well versed in the virtues of treating patients with special diets. Therefore, the options available to patients are narrow. For those with serious diseases, it's back to the drugs, surgery, and chemotherapy approach.

My only hope is that the new trend toward body awareness, and therefore more attention to dietary causes and cures, will help encourage a more organic approach to well-being.

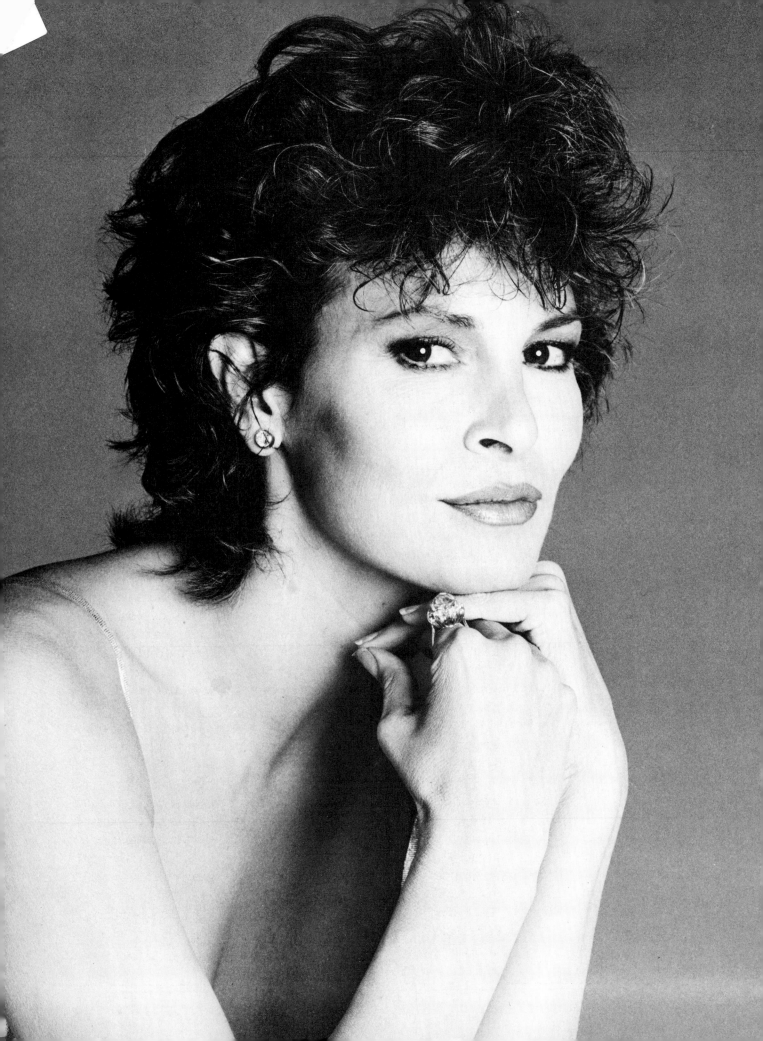

In Style

"**Style is being yourself, but on purpose.**"

Call it dash, chic, charisma—style is that indefinable quality that sets one apart from the herd. And like a fingerprint, it's unique, individual, and can't be faked.

There are no rules or special guidelines concerning style. Indeed, style is usually identified with someone who *breaks* the rules of conventional wisdom, not arbitrarily, but as a means of self-expression. Basically, it originates from doing what comes naturally. Or, as Quentin Crisp puts it, "Style is being yourself, but on purpose."

Who Are You?

Now, that can be a tricky question. Not only must you know precisely who you are, but you need the confidence to *show it*. And because to have style means to go out on a limb, most people shy away from expressing themselves too freely . . . afraid of letting something out of the closet. They opt for "playing it safe." To be sure, having style takes a fair degree of confidence and an extra amount of chutzpah!

Granted, you may want to edit your personality a bit for public consumption, but without pruning away or censoring all the idiosyncrasies that make you different from everyone else.

Which reminds me of some priceless words of advice given me by the late and great Italian director Vittorio de Sica. We were filming together in Rome, and at the time I was still groping for my own style. I knew people were interested in me primarily for my looks, and I was terribly self-conscious. Actually, I was simply anxious to please; and, given very little direction as an actress, I'd lost confidence.

Vittorio turned to me one day, smiled, and said, "My darling girl, please don't try to be perfect—*the defect is very important*." I never forgot it.

Style and the Academy Awards

In my profession, having style of one kind or another is a prerequisite. Sometimes it is even thought better to be considered plastic, tasteless, and vulgar than to have no style at all. So there are many types of "style" adopted by public figures, ranging from the sublime to the ridiculous.

Take, for example, the occasion of the annual Academy Awards. Here is an event where public "style" (or lack of it) is on display for all it is worth. And here is where approximately 400 million people, the world over, engage in the sport of separating the ones who have it from the ones that don't.

Over the years, I've appeared as a presenter on this televised extravaganza half a dozen times, with varying degrees of misgivings and success.

The first question asked of anyone who agrees to present an Oscar is, "What are you going to wear?" Whether or not this should be top priority is another question—the debate over the Awards show as a serious broadcast to honor artistic achievement versus the Academy Awards as a fashion show cum hype for the movie industry has never been resolved. I'd venture to say it's both. The fact remains that without a glamorous and exciting "style" of presentation, the Academy Awards would not be the same spectacular we've all come to know and love.

What to Wear

Chances are even the most faithful movie fan will not remember from one year to the next who won or lost, but they may recall down to the last detail what so-and-so was wearing! Deciding how to dress, then, can be an agonizing and excruciating task. Most attending actresses consider it the absolute pits! Some of us improve our stock with this brief appearance. Some go down for the count. Errors in judgment run rampant under pressure. Some are forgiven, some are not.

Undoubtedly, as far as "style" is concerned, the Academy Awards could be considered the *acid test*.

From Diane Keaton to Bette Midler

One famous costume designer offered these words of advice: "It's always best to look as tall and thin as possible." Well meaning though he was, he missed the mark. If he had his way, we would all show up looking safe, soignée, and boring, boring, boring. "Tall and thin"—meaning lots of black—is not always the answer. After all, it doesn't leave much room for scene stealers like Bette Midler or the refreshing eccentricity of a Diane Keaton. And who would we talk about after the show?

The truth is, there are no real rules in style. They are made

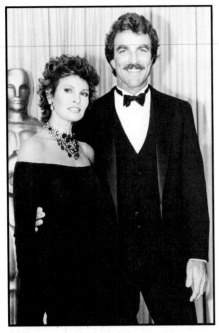

Above: *Getting my act together at the 1983 Oscars with Tom Selleck.*

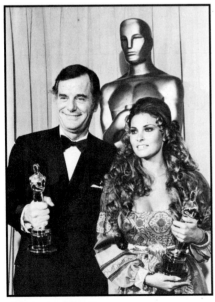

Above: *My first appearance on the Academy Awards, in 1970. I was described as "a barbecue queen at a Bar Mitzvah."*

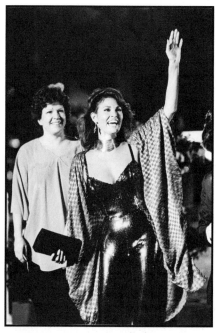

Above: *Blue-sequined jumpsuit, 1981. The trouble was I couldn't sit down in it!*

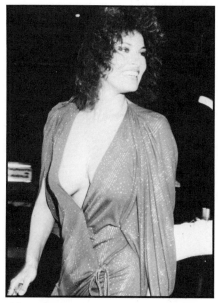

Above: *I've been told by the show's producers not to wear anything too tight or too low-cut. I haven't always obeyed.*

only to be broken. It's trial and error, hit or miss. If at first you don't succeed, try, try again—that is, if you get invited back the next time!

My first appearance on the Academy Awards, in 1970, had me qualify just under the wire. I was described as "a barbecue queen at a Bar Mitzvah." Not, as you may have guessed, quite the reaction I had hoped for . . . I had chosen a rather overblown creation with full sleeves and a Renaissance ballroom skirt in multicolored tapestry fabric. I should have known better than to venture forth that evening in a gown from a place called "Granny Takes a Trip"! But I was new at this.

In subsequent years, I appeared in considerably less yardage and with more favorable effect. Each year hence I've been told by the show's producers not to wear anything too tight or too low-cut. I haven't always obeyed.

One year, I decided to wear a skintight blue-sequined jumpsuit from my nightclub act that had proved to be a crowd pleaser. The only trouble was that, at the last minute, I found I couldn't sit down in it! (How was I to know? I always sang in the outfit standing up!) Eventually I had to unzip it and lie on my back in the limousine, all the way to the Dorothy Chandler Pavilion. Never again!

Another year, I wore a draped gown that was not tight-fitting but had a plunging neckline. That caused quite a stir, and I had to be careful how I moved. Several people forgot their dialogue that night because of it. I finally decided the best place for me was the backstage dressing room, where I could relax and wait until I was needed!

Regardless of the unintentional backstage comedy, I have finally managed to get my act together and develop a style that has served me well. It would have saved me a lot of wear and tear, however, had I known then what I know now.

The Clothesline

Clothes are an attitude. They should represent how you feel about yourself. Therefore, they should help lift your spirits if possible, instead of intimidating you. So don't let the clothes wear you; keep the upper hand. They can be alternately flamboyant or conservative, as long as they fit your mood, and the occasion. Clothes may make the first impression, but the lasting one depends on you.

Fashion Trends

Fashion is meant to influence and inspire you, but don't let it lead you around by the nose. You don't have to go along for the ride and become a "fashion victim" (haven't we all fallen into that

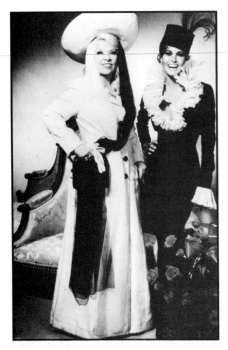

Above: *Mae West and I—a couple of fashion victims from* Myra Breckinridge, *1969.*

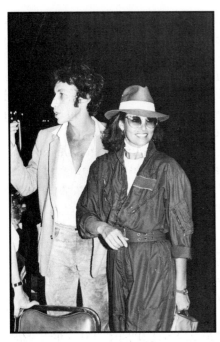

Above: *Caught traveling incognito in my army surplus flight suit.*

trap!). After all, it's *your* choice: you're the buyer. In the final analysis, it is you who dictate what is *in fashion* by exercising your prerogatives—not the other way around.

Budget

You don't need a lot of money to dress well or have style and class. In fact, more sins are committed against good taste by the nouveaux riches than by those who have to make choices based on budget limitations and practical need. Style is a common denominator; it breaks through social and economic barriers like a hot knife through butter. Anyone can have it.

Shopping

The best way I've found to shop is to stick to a designer I like and coordinate everything from one line of clothes. It keeps your style consistent, and *separates* tend to mix and match well. Barring that, a good boutique whose buyer has my taste is indispensable. Some department stores are beginning to coordinate things into boutique sections, so you can see what goes with what. If you had to buy a whole outfit running from one department to the next, you'd drop in your tracks!

Men's Clothes and Uniforms

I've always taken to men's clothes: jackets, hats, shirts, ties, vests, wristwatches. You name it, I've worn it. Many women's clothes today are heavily influenced by men's apparel. By contrast, the masculine touch accentuates our femininity and can prove quite sexy. Men's hats have dash on the female face. Dietrich, of course, caused a sensation in the thirties by donning naval-officer whites and men's suits. Uniforms, in particular, have a special message. They have their strength in numbers. Wearing one out of context brings to mind that strength, and it can be stunning on a woman.

For casual wear, I often go scavenging through army surplus shops for authentic flight suits, bomber jackets, etc. They're great for shopping around town, weekends, the country, and short trips to vacation spots. They are not, however, for everyone, on every occasion. You have to know what the traffic will bear. Somehow, I can't see Nancy Reagan in a paratrooper outfit, even on the weekend. Some people never let their hair down.

Dressing Down

A lot has been said about "dressing up," but very little about dressing down. Nobody should have every hair in place all the time, so don't neglect dressing for comfort. Put an outfit together on the spur of the moment that is charming, unassuming, and unpremeditated. No one likes a stuffed shirt. It's not much fun to be one either.

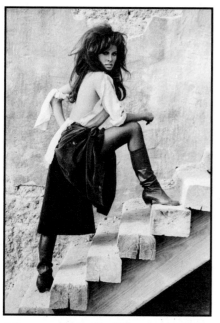

Above: *Nobody likes a stuffed shirt.* Bandolero *with James Stewart and Dean Martin (1968).*

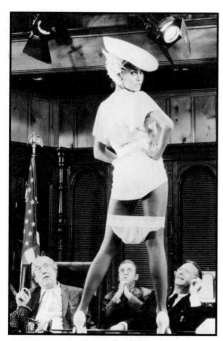

Above: *Dressing down in* Myra Breckinridge *could be a risky business. Here my composure sort of slipped.*

Being in the public eye, I found myself worrying far too much about what to wear to this and that everyday sortie about town. It got to the point where I didn't want to go to the corner drugstore without being dressed to kill. I got over it.

My favorite outfit now is a pair of worn-in blue jeans, a T-shirt with a sweatshirt thrown over it, old socks, sneakers, and a soft scarf, and I'm happy as a clam. No kidding. If I have to go out, I slip into a man-sized trench coat, add another scarf, grab my man's cap, and I'm out the door. I used to dread that people would recognize me without my movie-star drag—but they don't seem to mind; in fact, they seem more friendly that way on the streets. After all, there's a time for heavy-duty, drop-dead glamour and a time for relaxed easygoing dressing. You can look good too in your cozy clothes. People will wanna "cozy up" to ya.

Inverse Snobbery

I love clothes. I also love people who hate them. Unwittingly, they make fashion more important. Fashion has gotten a bad name in some circles because it's perceived as something designed to make an existing wardrobe obsolete. But you could say the same thing about cars, weapons, young girls, and electronics! Of course, the price tags on some retail merchandise—not to mention couture collections—are just outrageous. It drives a girl to basic black.

Fashion Design

Fashion designers create by observing the natural instincts of unself-conscious people in practical situations. It's surprising to note that some of the world's top designers are heavily influenced by the way the peasants, farmers, or fishermen of various countries layer their clothing, tie their scarves, drape their bodies, and combine colors, fabrics, and accessories. So never feel that you need be unduly "sophisticated" to be stylish.

I'm not suggesting you wear a folk-dancing costume to meet with your banker, but there's always something in everyone's background or way of living that is the key to his or her personal style. So take the time to look for it.

Playing Around

Playing, especially for grown-ups, is essential. But it is particularly stimulating for someone who is developing a style. Go to the theater, read a good book, listen to music, wander through flea markets, thumb through history books, and browse through museums. Above all, daydream. These are not trivial pastimes. They are a means of making connections and of gathering inspiration. You can't invent anything of any consequence without them—much less yourself.

Beauty

Hair is a sensitive subject. It says who we are faster than our credit card. It's the easiest way to spot a person's hang-ups. And for that reason it is probably the most overdone and overdesigned part of our appearance.

Hairstyle

Fussing with our hair is a favorite pastime. We fluff it, swirl it, curl and blow it, we pat it, slick it, tie it, braid and color it. But nothing is as crucial as the way we *cut* it.

Men and women alike live in fear of the haircut that will open them up to ridicule and embarrassment. There's nothing worse than having someone shear your ears and neck so that they stick out like a sore thumb. It's humiliating. Which is maybe why the army does it to recruits the first minute it lays hands on them. Nothing can cut you down to size more than a bad haircut. *That's why I cut my own.* That way, if I make a mistake, I've got no one else to blame.

There's nothing worse than having someone shear your ears and neck so that they stick out like a sore thumb.

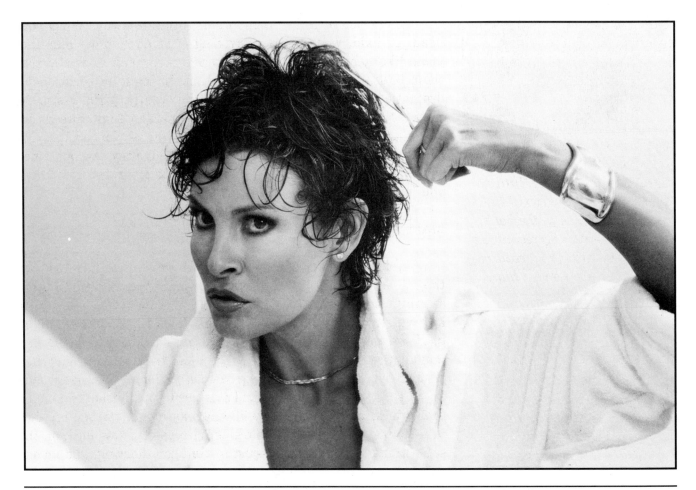

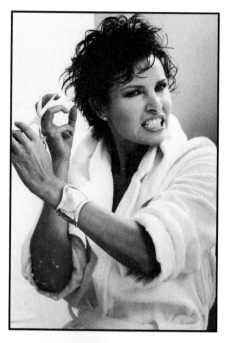

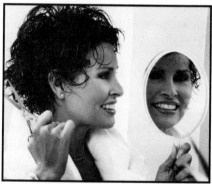

Opposite and above: *Trim your hair slightly where you want it to look fuller. Cutting adds height on the top of the head and volume to the back and sides. With this technique you can balance your features (check your profile in a hand mirror).*

In over fifteen years of professional life, I've known very few good haircutters. I'm not speaking of hair *stylists,* who can make even a bad cut look good—there are a number of them in the fashion and movie business who are superb. But down-to-the-nitty-gritty, the important thing is *cutting* talent. And that is rare.

Besides, I hate to be bullied around by someone I've never seen before, or put myself in the hands (or at the mercy) of a total stranger right before an important commitment. So I cut it myself.

Besides, when I'm on location shooting, or performing eight shows a week on Broadway, I haven't the time to get to a salon; and my favorite cutters are left behind. So I cut it myself!

It's not that I'm especially brave—or even stubborn—but out of necessity I've learned how to do it. Besides, short hair is easy. When I first cut my long hair short, three years ago, it took me a whole week. I cut it little by little each day, gaining confidence with each swipe of the scissors. For the back, I used an additional mirror, on a stand. I enjoyed designing the shape on my own. It taught me a lot about myself. So if you are ready for a change, or want to take matters into your own hands—if only on occasion, when you're stuck on your own, why don't you try it?

Hair Spray

Unless you're a TV anchorman, throw it away! Wrap your head, go bald, wear a hat—anything—but don't have hair that looks like a helmet. It's hard to convince women and men that their hair should *move!* You can slick it down on occasion for dramatic effect or use gels for body; but really, girls, resist the urge to make beehives, lampshades, gondolas, or tumbleweeds out of your hair! It's inexcusable, unless, of course, you are playing the clown. Clowns are very nice people—but they are not taken seriously. If the purpose is to get a laugh, be my guest. But I hope you have a *paying* audience.

Makeup

My first experience in a Hollywood makeup department, for the movie *Fantastic Voyage,* was a real shocker. I found myself staring into a mirror at a total stranger—I looked like a powder keg with two eyes and a pair of lips! The makeup man swore he used the same technique on me that, back in the "old days," had made Linda Darnell into a star. But I had the sneaking suspicion that, although we were shooting in Technicolor, I'd just been made up for a black-and-white movie! I muttered a quick thanks, jumped into my car, drove like crazy all the way home, washed my face in a frenzy, and redid the whole thing myself. I was back on the set—minus the white stuff—just in time for shooting; and no one said a word.

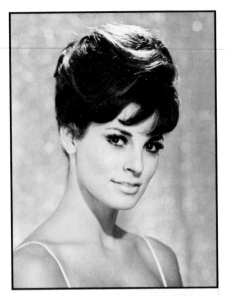

Above: *As a deb star in 1964, I was given a screen test at 20th Century-Fox.*

I can remember back when I stuck on three pairs of eyelashes at a time! It was the style. But now, when I look at those photos, I can't believe I had the guts to do it.

The next day, I was called into the front office. "Just who do you think you are?" demanded Dick Zanuck, the head of the studio, no less. All I managed to say was, "I don't want to look like Linda Darnell." "So you think you know more than the experts?" he countered. "No," I said, "but I want to look like myself, and I think I'm the best expert on that subject." Fortunately, he seemed to accept my plea, told me he liked my spirit, and we became friends.

The poor makeup artist who did me the first day never came near me again. He handed me a powder puff and told me I was on my own; and, like the man said, I have been ever since.

Of course, I owe a debt to many talented makeup artists over the years, who have added refinements, pointed out errors, taught me about lighting, and watched and protected me "on camera" as no one else could; and to them I am eternally grateful.

At any rate, I learned a lot and did become an expert, so to speak. I take pride in the fact that I've made myself pretty independent in that department, and I'm happy to share some of the tricks of the trade with you.

Tricks of My Trade

There are three main concerns in doing a great makeup. The first is that less is more. Always use the minimum amount you can get away with, for the maximum effect. Makeup that shouts at you is no good at all. The second is that highlighting and shadowing should be used to accentuate the positive and eliminate the negative. Obviously, this technique works best when your makeup is perfectly blended so that your face doesn't look like it's been painted by the numbers. The third is to always consider the light you're going to be seen in, since it will affect your choice of colors.

1. Less Is More. I can remember back when I stuck on three pairs of eyelashes at a time! It was the style. But now, when I look at those photos, I can't believe I had the guts to do it. Oh, well, everything is relative, and we're all influenced by the times. But they keep changing. If you get good at doing your face, your makeup should change with them. So your face won't get left behind as the years go by.

2. Accentuate the Positive, Eliminate the Negative. Everyone uses makeup primarily to correct something about their features they don't like, so they can put their best face forward. Accentuating the positive and eliminating the negative involves the technique of highlighting and shadowing.

For example, by highlighting a line down the top of your nose and shadowing the sides, you can make it appear narrower. Shadowing just at the tip makes it appear shorter. By experimenting with this technique you can modify or accentuate the shape of any feature, including the cheekbones, chin, eyes, and jawline.

Only the best restaurants have beautiful soft lighting, while most offices sport the harsh green flicker of fluorescent tubing. It's enough to turn you into Godzilla.

3. Lighting and Color. One thing I have learned from being photographed under a wide variety of conditions is that makeup is only as good as the light it's seen in. So you have to compensate for the existing lighting in any surrounding.

There are times when the daylight is slate gray—bluish in tone—with less warm, peachy, flattering shades. The better the light, the better we look. But, alas, the romantic days of candlelight are over! Only the best restaurants have beautiful soft lighting, while most offices sport the harsh green flicker of fluorescent tubing. It's enough to turn you into Godzilla.

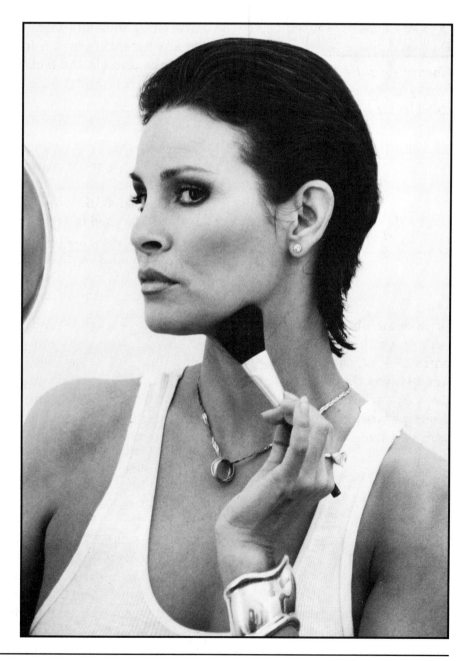

Right: *I learned to mix and match makeup on my face, much as a painter mixes colors on his palette. Here, applying blusher.*

So it's best to keep lighting conditions in mind while making up, to compensate for bad lighting, to avoid aggravating an unflattering situation or clashing with existing light. Under difficult conditions, certain shades of red will tend to "read" too darkly on the lips and cheeks, and too much bronze in your foundation can look muddy. I've found it's best to use a lighter touch and stick to clearer colors.

Generally speaking, at night, in dimly lit surroundings, you can afford to go for a more dramatic look. For daytime, a more natural, subtle makeup is better. Just being aware of the light is all that's necessary to temper your choice of colors and the amount of makeup you wear on any given occasion.

I always try to make up at a window for bright sunlight and in artificial light for evenings or dark days. I like to strike a happy medium between inside lighting and outside daylight. For professional appearances I use a classic dressing-room type of makeup mirror to simulate the bright lights around the cameras.

Below: *A professional makeup kit makes me into a one-man band.*

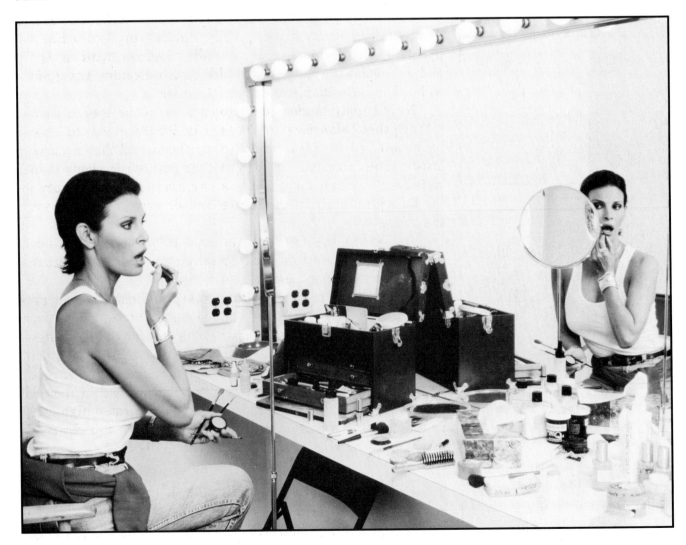

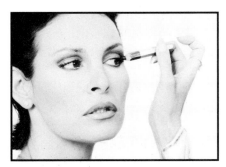

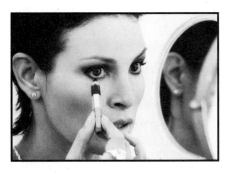

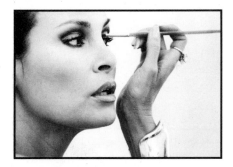

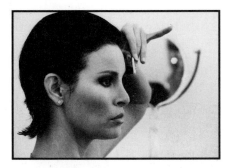

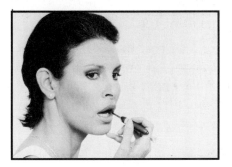

One of a Kind

Since each of us is unique, I would not presume to tell you how to *do* your face. Also, because makeup is part of your style, you should develop it yourself. But if you're curious, here's how I do my own face, along with an explanation of the techniques I use:

1. Moisturizer. I apply moisturizer to my face and neck before I begin. Give it a chance to sink in. I use one that works under makeup, not a thick heavy night cream. If your skin is oily, perhaps you don't need one, as there is already some moisturizer in most makeup.

2. Eyes. I always do my eyes first, as a morale booster. Then, if I don't have time for the rest, at least I have an expressive face. The eyes are the windows to the soul, they say.

First I curl my lashes and apply mascara. I dust the lashes with powder before a second application of mascara; it makes them thicker.

Then I apply *liner* under the eye next to the lashes and extend it past the outer corner, gracefully slanting up. I also line the upper lid, the outside corner only. Smudge with a Q-Tip and powder with a small powder brush (square tip, ½-inch wide). This helps to blend and set the liner.

Next I apply *shadow* to the top portion of the eyelids. I make a shape that balances with the liner under the eyes, and I blend it upward and outward, first with my finger and then a makeup brush. (The brush I keep for just that purpose is about ½-inch wide, small enough to get into this area gracefully.) Then I powder the lid with a medium-size, barrel-shaped powder brush (I avoid the lashes).

A special touch is to add an extra color—blue or mauve or burgundy—just under the liner, creating an iridescent effect that softens the look. Don't forget to blend.

For special occasions, to bring sweep and dash to your eyes, it's fun to add lashes to the outside corner of your own upper lashes. Or cut up strip lashes and use the pieces to fill in wherever your own are missing. It takes more time and patience, but it's effective. Apply with tweezers and lash adhesive. This works best with lashes that are already made with alternating thin and thick sections. Also for evenings, I sometimes add a frosted highlighter in soft pastel, ever so lightly, on the eyelid, between the crease and the upper lashes. But only in the center above the iris—otherwise you could look like a raccoon.

3. Application. Everything must be blended. No harsh lines, and don't stop at the chin. That's not easy, especially if you have to rise at 5:00 A.M. and slap on the pan stick at 6:00 A.M., as I often

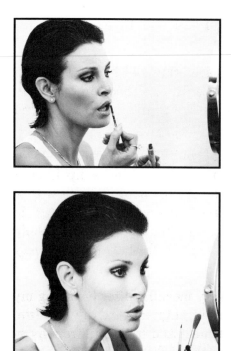

do. Blend down the neck a little and don't forget your eyelids. I use a small sponge or my fingertips.

4. Foundation. A foundation color must blend with your skin tone and enhance it. Try some on the inside of your wrist first, as a test. Your face is always lighter than the rest of your body. It's supposed to be. Even if you're very tan, your face and neck should be a few shades lighter than the rest of you.

5. Highlighter. For highlighting, select a shade lighter than your base, but one that blends with your foundation in color and texture. Since it goes in the delicate area under the eyes and around the nose and mouth, it should be a light consistency, not too heavy, or it will accentuate wrinkles. Testing is the only way to determine this.

Apply under the eyes with fingertips or brush and blend outward all the way past the corner of the eyes above the cheekbones. Apply also around the nostrils, under the nose, and in the creases from your nose to the corners of the mouth if you need it. Blend perfectly with fingertips and makeup brush. Powder with fluffy large powder brush.

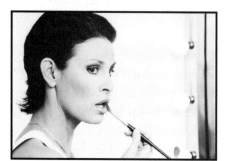

6. Powder. Most people powder at the end of their foundation, after applying highlighting and shadowing, blusher, etc. As for me, I powder as I go along. When I finish an area, I dust it lightly with powder. It's very unorthodox, but it assures me that all my careful effort won't get smudged. I'm a perfectionist. By the time I'm finished, my moisturizer has already started to shine through. Since I have a dry complexion, this keeps me from having that "powder keg" look which, as you know by now, I've never liked and never will. I always use a loose translucent powder, and sometimes I dab over it with rose water on a damp piece of cotton.

7. Blusher. I apply my creme blusher over powdered cheeks to bring back shine. But it takes a very delicate touch. It can also be done before you powder. I use a coral color and start under my cheekbones and blend up and in with my fingertips, so that I have faint roses on my cheeks from full front. I also blend blusher onto my temples, forehead, chin tip, and jawline. Then dust with powder once again. It's also nice on the brow bone, just under the outer sweep of your brows.

Sometimes I use a yellow blusher over the tips of cheeks, forehead, and jaw; it can give a peachy glow.

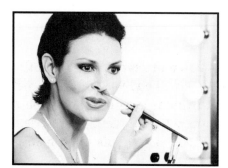

You may want to add more powder blush to this, or leave it alone. Sometimes I do, sometimes I don't. It depends on my mood and where I'm going.

8. Cheekbones. I shadow very lightly with a taupe-brown color

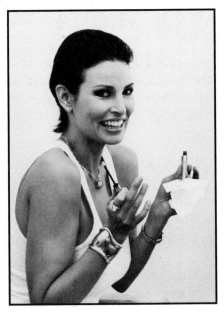

Above: *A smile supplies the finishing touch!*

I know that when I feel good, I look good—and no amount of makeup or clothes can give me that!

under my cheekbones. Easy does it. I love David Bowie, but that's not the effect I'm going for!

9. Eyebrows. I fill in only the places that need it—painted-on brows are artificial looking. Use a pencil one shade lighter than your color. Powder away the shine. Use a clean lash brush to blend pencil strokes.

10. Lips. I always put lip balm on first. Then I add my basic lipstick color from the tube and blot. Next, using a lip liner, I outline the shape of my mouth, and fill in the difference with a lipstick brush. Then I blot the edges and use a much lighter lip liner to go over the first one to soften it; then I powder just the lip line, which softens it further, and apply a frosted lip gloss, very sparingly.

11. Eye Drops. I use eye drops every morning after brushing my teeth. I think they are a great beauty treatment, and my eyes love them. They help to soothe away dryness and irritation from overheating or tiredness. I use the kind that takes the red out so that I don't have road maps in my eyes over the breakfast table. But if your eyes are sensitive, I recommend you consult your eye doctor.

Gilding the Lily

I've often thought that it would be nice if we could all look like a million every day. It would help a lot in my business, where I'm on display much of the time. But I know that when I feel good, I look good—and no amount of makeup or clothes can give me that!

The more you exercise and watch your weight, the less makeup you'll need. I've found it to be true that when I'm "in training," my face glows with health and I hate to cover it up with makeup. By the same token, for occasions when makeup is a must, it goes on much better over a healthy complexion.

After all is said and done, glowing health is the best beauty treatment!

Stylishly Fit

In the final analysis, style boils down to developing a healthy mind in a healthy body. If you feel good about yourself, the rest seems to follow. So the purpose of all this is simply to give you a glimpse of the possibilities that are open to you when you pursue a regular program, such as this method, that builds and ensures *total* beauty and fitness.

Writing on My Own / Unborrowed Opinions

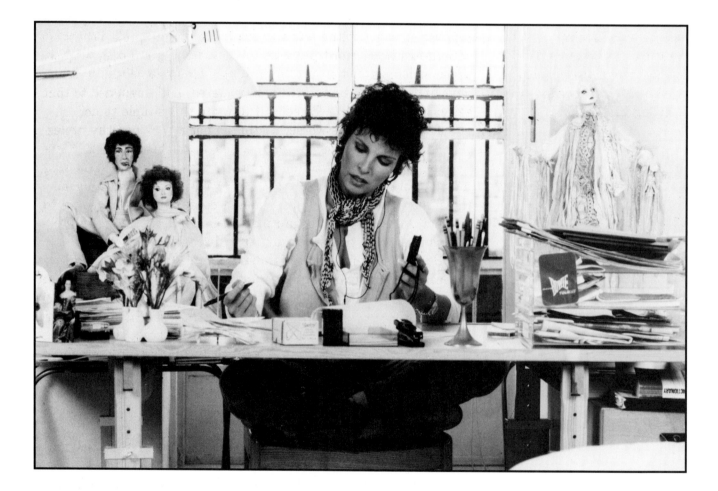

To sit down and write a book alone was a brand-new experience for me, and looking back on it, I'm amazed that I undertook such an awesome task in the first place. It has been one of the most stimulating and at the same time exasperating experiences I've ever had. In my role as first-time writer, I found myself stumbling along in a hopelessly naïve fashion, often brushing dangerously close to disaster. Fortunately, I managed to land on my feet each time just on the eve of a deadline.

> When it got to the point where I was having profane conversations with my word processor, I realized I was going slightly bananas.

The first period was positively exhilarating . . . a totally euphoric feeling of writing away each morning at my desk overlooking the Manhattan skyline. I thought this was the ultimate luxury—self-expression in its purest form, with no one else's reactions to get in the way, nobody to tell me what to do, nobody to ask permission of and compromise with, and nobody to . . . well, absolutely nobody!

It was alright for a while to be away from the ballyhoo of show business, but eventually these bouts of writer's solitude started to wear on me, and I began looking around for an opinion—any opinion. When it got to the point where I was having profane conversations with my word processor, I realized I was going slightly bananas. I was lost in a labyrinth of words and ideas, of delete keys and insert buttons. What, I wondered, had happened to that self-possessed person who set out to write this simple tome?

To make matters worse, writing is not a very healthy profession, especially for someone doing a health and beauty book. Nothing before had ever broken down my fitness resolve—not making movies, not television, not Broadway or Vegas. But, suddenly, now the sight of an empty legal pad and a cupful of pens drove me to the point of cracking. I began playing hooky from my daily exercise routine and stuffing myself with chocolate chip cookies!

But the most frightening thing of all was to discover that after several months of writing like crazy, there simply wasn't enough room to say all the things I had in mind.

Writing this book was absolutely cathartic. Suddenly, with pen in hand, the dam was bursting on every subject imaginable, from the battle of the sexes to foreign policy. I found myself going off on tangents. For instance, when writing about building strength and the use of force for physical fitness, I was making comparisons to missile deployments and the American military policy in Central America and the Middle East. Try as I might to stifle myself, it was to no avail. I was stricken with a case of socio-political influenza.

I kept telling myself, "Come on, Rocky, this is *just* a health and beauty book," but I had a hard time convincing myself that there was anything trivial about the subject, and I still do. On the contrary, it's basic to our state of being, and eventually to the world at large. Encouraged by this rationale, I penned volumes of unborrowed opinions on the changing image of America, the upcoming Presidential elections, the low priority given to education, medical care, and public transportation, and the disenchantment with leadership in an era of mediocrity. All, mind you, neatly interwoven through the green beans and the Wonder Soup, or tucked away discreetly between flexibility and the central nervous system.

Finally, I came to my senses and for the sake of style and the sanity of my publisher, who politely referred to these detours as "too didactic," I managed to edit myself for public consumption. But not without first reexamining why I had set out on this odyssey to begin with.

It wasn't to talk about how it feels to turn forty, or how to stay young forever so that in old age you can fade away into the sunset looking like nineteen from the rear end. Of course, I wanted to help people look and feel better about themselves. But more importantly, I sought to offer an alternative to the current trends in fitness.

Fitness *is* an important issue today. In a time when all of us realize that much of what happens, on a larger scale, is outside of our control, we've turned to ourselves to make the best of our own individual lives, where we *can* make a difference and effect real change. Fitness is indeed a political movement—a new twist on the demonstrations of the sixties. When 20,000 people jog together through the streets of some of our major cities, it is without a doubt their bid for a better world!

I also think there is a relationship between how people prepare for fitness and their general philosophy of life. Some approach it as though they were preparing for combat, like soldiers at boot camp—the old drill-instructor approach. On the other hand, this book represents a nonviolent approach. Although I concede that there's room for both, my preference is for the latter, because, in the final analysis, it defuses the fear and anxiety that make a combative approach necessary.

I'm no namby-pamby and I'm prepared to do battle for something I believe in. But not when there are better ways available to get the same results. This book was the smallest soapbox I could find to stand on. But the message is loud and clear. Violence breeds violence! Let's put a stop to it in every way we can. It could all start with us!

When 20,000 people jog together through the streets of some of our major cities, it is without a doubt their bid for a better world.

Acknowledgments

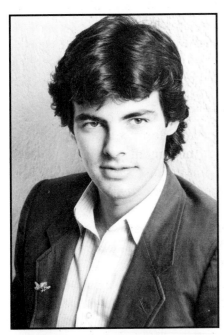

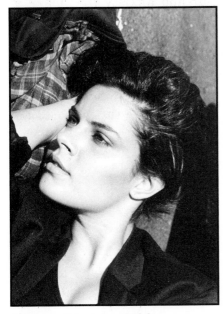

Above: *My two children— Damon, 24, and Tahnee, 22. The latest editions.*

As an actress weaned on those epic award-ceremony speeches, I couldn't pass up this opportunity to get sentimental over everyone near and dear to me during the course of this book. My love and thanks go to the following people:

Damon, my son—for being supportive, protective, sensitive, and understanding.

Tahnee, my daughter—for being both beautiful and bright and my best friend.

My mom, Jo—for being herself. She's inspirational!

My sister and brother, Gayle and Jim—who both practice yoga on the West Coast.

My dad, Armand—because I know he'd be proud of me.

B.J. Ward—my L.A. friend and the one who introduced me to this method.

Jerry Harvey—my long-distance buddy who sympathized.

Eileen Poole—my nutritionist and confidante.

Rochelle Udell—my barometer of style and taste. The only mellow person left in New York City.

Dick Seaver, my editor at Holt, Rinehart and Winston—for his enthusiasm in the project and his confidence in me.

Jane Pasanen, Pat Breinin, Bob Reed, Karen Gillis, Jack Macrae, Karen Mender, David Stanford, and everyone at Holt who worked daily on this book.

Trent Duffy—my production editor and morale booster.

Eliane Laffont—a real life dynamo. For all her savvy.

Marc Stein and George Slaff—my attorneys and friends, who both stepped out of a Frank Capra movie.

All my yoga teachers over the years: Alan Finger, Bill Porter, Jacqui Davis, Moya Devi, Mark Becker, Evelyn Brooks, and last but not least Bikram Choudhury, who was my first teacher and who most influenced my daily practice until this day.

And a special thanks to Chat, our dog. The first nonviolent Doberman, who warmed my feet under the table on many a late night.

Without these people and one dog, this book could never have happened.

Photo Credits

All photographs are by André Weinfeld, with the following exceptions:

Vera Anderson: p. 263 (top).
Author's collection: pp. viii, 7, 14, 16.
Bunte Magazine: p. 242 (bottom).
Elle Magazine/Tony Kent/Sygma: p. 242 (top).
Film Export AG/Terry O'Neill: pp. 19, 216.
Films Christian Fechner: p. 10.
Tim Geany: p. 263 (bottom).
Hammer Film Productions Ltd.: p. 6.
Harper's Bazaar © 1982 The Hearst Corporation/Francesco Scavullo: p. 236 (bottom).
Henson Associates: p. 221.
Tony Kent/Sygma: pp. 8 (top), 23, 27 (left and top middle), 28–29, 231 (top middle), 264.
Tony Kent/Sygma/RWP Inc: pp. 226 (right), 227 (bottom right), 236 (top).
Tony Kent/copyright © 1979 by *Playboy:* p. iv (reproduced by special permission of *Playboy* Magazine).
Jean Pierre Laffont/Sygma: pp. 24 (bottom), 260.
Harry Langdon: pp. 9, 15, 231 (top right).
Life Magazine/André Weinfeld: p. 237 (bottom) (courtesy *Life* Picture Service).
Los Angeles Magazine/Claude Mougin: p. 233.
Los Angeles Times/copyright © 1979/1983 *Los Angeles Times:* pp. 248 (top), 249 (top).
MGM/UA: p. 11 (top) © 1972 Metro-Goldwyn-Mayer Inc.
Terry O'Neill/Woodfin Camp & Associates: pp. 11 (bottom), 18 (bottom).
Robin Platzer/Images: p. 250 (bottom).
Playbill/Francesco Scavullo: p. 237 (top) (*Playbill* is a registered trademark of Playbill Inc., New York, used by permission).
Morgan Renard/American International Pictures, © 1974: p. 220 (by permission of Orion Pictures Corporation).
Roma's Press Photo: p. 4 (by permission).
Francesco Scavullo: p. 246.
Eva Sereny/*Playboy Guide:* pp. 1 (all), 2 (all), 3 (all).
Eva Sereny/Sygma: pp. 18 (top), 27 (top right), 230 (top left), 231 (bottom middle), 235 (top).
Sipa Special Features: p. 249 (bottom).
Skrebneski: p. 215 (by permission).
Alice Springs: p. 12.
Stern Magazine: p. 244 (bottom).
Rene Techer: p. 24 (top).
Time Magazine © 1969 Time Inc. All rights reserved: p. 234 (top) (reprinted by permission from *Time*).
20th Century-Fox: pp. 20, 250 (top), 251 (both).
United Press International: p. 248 (bottom).
Chris Von Wangenheim/RWP Inc: pp. 225, 228–29.
Chris Von Wangenheim/copyright © 1979 by *Playboy:* p. 235 (bottom) (reproduced by special permission of *Playboy* Magazine).
Woman's Own Magazine/Harry Langdon: p. 244 (top).
Zodiac Productions: p. 254.

Below: *André—a true Renaissance man.*

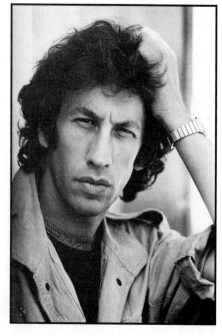

All photographs by André Weinfeld, including the jacket photograph, were taken with a Hasselblad 500 EL/M camera equipped with Carl Zeiss 80mm, 150mm, and 250mm lenses.

Ms. Welch's hair by Odile for Bruno/Dessange, New York.

Front jacket jewelry by Bulgari.